..RET COLLEGE
.. CAMPUS LIBRARY

Growing Up with a Chronic Disease
The Impact on Children and their Families

e stamped below

QUEEN MARGARET COLLEGE LIBRARY

of related interest

Interventions with Bereaved Children
Edited by Susan C. Smith and Sister Margaret Pennells
ISBN 1 85302 285 3

Children with Special Needs
Assessment, Law and Practice – Caught in the Acts, 3rd Edition
John Friel
ISBN 1 85302 280 2

Young Adults with Special Needs
Assessment, Law and Practice – Caught in the Acts
John Friel
ISBN 1 85302 231 4

Community Care Practice and the Law
Michael Mandelstam with Belinda Schwer
ISBN 1 85302 273 X

Growing Up with a Chronic Disease
The Impact on Children and their Families

Christine Eiser

Jessica Kingsley Publishers
London and Bristol, Pennsylvania

All rights reserved. No paragraph of this publication may be reproduced, copied or transmitted save with written permission or in accordance with the provisions of the Copyright Act 1956 (as amended), or under the terms of any licence permitting limited copying issued by the Copyright Licensing Agency, 33–34 Alfred Place, London WC1E 7DP.

Any person who does any unauthorised act in relation to this publication may be liable to criminal prosecution and civil claims for damages.

The right of Christine Eiser to be identified as author of this work has been asserted by her in accordance with the Copyright, Designs and Patents Act 1988.

First published in the United Kingdom in 1993 by
Jessica Kingsley Publishers Ltd
116 Pentonville Road
London N1 9JB
and
1900 Frost Road, Suite 101
Bristol, PA 19007, USA

Second impression 1995

Copyright © 1993 Christine Eiser

British Library Cataloguing in Publication Data
Eiser, Christine
Growing up with a Chronic Disease:
The Impact on Children and their Families
I. Title
155.9

ISBN 1-85302-168-7

Printed and Bound in Great Britain by
Athenaeum Press, Gateshead, Tyne and Wear

Contents

Preface

The idea for this book came from a belief that psychological work has a contribution to make toward the total care of children with chronic diseases, but that this contribution was so far so small as to be almost negligible. Although the quantity of relevant work has increased enormously during the last decade, most of it languishes in academic psychology journals, and is not even read by practising medical staff. Sometimes psychologists themselves seem unaware of the potential practical relevance of their work. This book is not an exhaustive review of available literature, but I have attempted to focus on that which is of more immediate practical value. I have also tried to identify issues which have failed to attract the attention that they deserve.

This work was primarily funded by a grant from the Leverhulme Trust, to whom I am deeply indebted. I have also drawn heavily on examples from empirical research which has been funded by other bodies, including the E.S.R.C., the M.R.C., the Northcott Devon Medical Foundation, the University of Exeter Research Fund and the Cancer Research Campaign.

I would like to thank all my colleagues in Exeter for their help and support over the years, and especially Trudy Havermans. Much of this book was written while visiting Carleton University, Ottawa in Canada, and I am especially grateful to them for the opportunity to work in such an attractive environment. I thank especially Jan Gordon-Walker for long research discussions. I would also like to thank my Australian friends, Penny Cousens, Daphne Glaun and Heather Mohay, for their advice and encouragement. Finally, I should acknowledge Dick, David and Ben.

Overview

The first three chapters of this book describe the impact of chronic disease on the child during three stages of development; infancy and the pre-school period, middle childhood and adolescence. It is emphasised that there are unique stressors associated with chronic disease as a function of these different developmental periods. Essentially, during the infancy and pre- school period, it is very difficult for the child to understand the seriousness of the disease, or to anticipate the long-term aspects of treatment. Treatment is, of course, the responsibility of the parents. Central issues are likely to involve achieving cooperation from such a young child, especially where these are so much at odds with the child's preferred life-style. (At these ages, children like to eat when they are hungry or feel like eating. Children with diabetes will be encouraged to eat at regular times, whether they are hungry or not; those with cystic fibrosis will be encouraged to eat more than they would otherwise choose since the disease involves a breakdown in the body's ability to metabolise foods efficiently). Confrontation between parent and child is likely over everyday care-taking tasks, especially feeding and disciplining.

During the middle-school period, the child begins to demand some independence from the family, and spends more time in the company of peers. Chronic disease poses a challenge to school-life and academic achievements. The need for regular treatment and hospital visits disrupts school attendance, with some adverse consequences for academic success and peer relationships. Through meetings and social interactions with peers, children with chronic disease are forced to recognise differences between themselves and others, sometimes with deleterious consequences for self-esteem.

During adolescence, responsibility for self-care is shifted systematically on to the individual, and parents' role is reduced to one of occasional surveillance. Adolescents must find ways of explaining the disease to others and find new friendship groups away from home. Depending on the nature of the disease, some adolescents must come to terms with restrictions on work or social opportunities, and acknowledge reduced fertility or limited life-expectancy.

Although the potential impact of chronic disease can be understood from such a developmental perspective, it is also apparent from these reviews that the characteristic response of many children is one of resilience and survival rather than trauma and maladjustment. The traditional assumption that psychopathology is the common response to chronic disease in children is not substantiated. There is an anomaly in that much research has focussed on the negative consequences of chronic disease, and individuals are often given little opportunity to describe their strengths and coping resources. In contrast, recent theoretical models stress the likelihood of normal growth and development, even in the face of serious and life-threatening disease. These approaches are reviewed in Chapter 5. Again a developmental theme is identified; the appraisal of stress and available coping strategies are a function of the child's chronological age. Mothers and fathers also differ in their perceptions of the stresses associated with disease, and tend to adopt predictably different methods of coping. Again reflecting the developmental theme in the child, family and disease, it is apparent that choice of coping strategies is also a function of the stage in disease progression. Although this work points to the relative value of some coping strategies over others, there is no evidence to suggest that any one coping style will be universally superior; what works for some people in some circumstances will not necessarily work for others.

While the impact of chronic disease is partly dependent on developmental factors, the influence of the family is critical at all stages. For this reason, in the remaining chapters, chronic childhood disease as experienced by other family members is considered. Mothers and fathers differ in their perceptions of the seriousness and impact of the disease; in their responsibility for disease management, and their own psychological reactions to the problem. Fathers appear more stoic, take on greater responsibility for other children in the family and often cope by throwing themselves into their work defining their role as the family breadwinner. This role is also protective, in that interactions with the sick child and hospital personnel is minimised. In contrast, mothers bear the brunt of responsibility for home-treatments, and spend more time with the sick child compared with fathers. This throws them into greater contact with medical staff and leads to greater knowledge of the disease process and prognosis. The outcome seems to be associated with a differential impact on parents' mental health, with mothers showing more anxiety and depression, as well as physical ill-health. Chronic disease has also been linked with increases in marital strain and sometimes increased probability of separation and divorce. Evidence for these claims is considered in Chapter 6, as well as the implications of parents' mental health and marital relations for the child's functioning.

Having a child with chronic disease raises some basic questions about the goals of parenting. Parents who previously felt it was very important that the child succeed academically may wish to re-evaluate these ideals when the child's life seems threatened. Or they may come to value the here-and-now, and place greater value on simply being with the child. Parents who had clear ideas about family discipline may find these challenged by the need to balance the child's wishes with restrictions that are associated with the disease. It is possible, for example, for parents to believe that 14-year-olds are generally capable of getting up early to do a paper-round and need to learn how to budget their own finances, but worry that the 14-year-old with diabetes may consequently have too little time to attend conscientiously to treatment management. In these circumstances, parents face some conflict between their basic beliefs about parenting and their knowledge that time must be allowed before school for adequate testing of blood sugar and insulin injections. Chapter 7 is concerned with issues such as these, and reviews the work concerned with the consequences of chronic disease for parenting.

The same theme is continued and extended in Chapter 8, with the emphasis on the relation between parenting and the child's response to treatment. Families may be instrumental in promoting good adjustment to disease management by providing a home environment in which the child is well placed to learn about the disease and become responsible for self-care. Alternatively, they can make it more difficult for the child to accept treatment or come to terms with the implications of the disease by challenging the authority or expertise of medical staff, or questioning the value of treatment. The interdependence between the child's adjustment and family functioning is emphasised.

It is often said that healthy siblings are the biggest losers in any family where one child has a chronic illness. Parents are typically occupied by the needs of the sick child. In a mistaken belief that they are protecting healthy siblings from unnecessary anxiety, parents can appear to exclude these children from much family activity. The naivity of this approach is seen whenever siblings themselves are allowed to speak about their experiences. Many are acutely aware of the crisis, and lack of opportunity to talk to parents increases, rather than reduces, their anxiety. In Chapter 9, the impact of chronic disease on healthy siblings is considered as it affects cognitive, social and emotional development. Greater attention needs to be given to siblings' concerns, both for their own benefit, and also because they can play a crucial role in facilitating good adjustment in the sick child.

In the final chapter, the focus is on defining the psychologist's role in caring for the sick child. Good care is dependent on a team approach, and this can be problematic given differences in training of the various health professions. The role of the psychologist in caring for the sick child is changing and must continue to change. In the past, the emphasis was on dealing with the dying child, and helping families through the bereavement period. With improvements in treatments of a range of chronic conditions, the need is now to help children *live* with chronic disease. The limitations of psychopathological models are continuously apparent and the need for more coping orientated models clear. This must now also be reflected in research and intervention strategies. The role of the psychologist is increasingly moving in the direction of health promotion, with an emphasis on education, prevention of difficulties, and minimisation of the impact of chronic disease on normal growth and development.

CHAPTER 1

Chronic Disease
The Nature of the Challenge

In an age and culture in which good health is taken for granted, parents expect their children to be well and survive them. Diseases which threaten children's autonomy and compromise their life-expectancy challenge our emotions and coping resources to their limits. Childhood disease can turn the world upside down.

Yet these challenges are faced by a sizeable population. Some 10–15% of children under 16 years of age are affected by chronic, long-term conditions (Cadman, Boyle, Szatmari & Offord 1987; Rutter, Tizard & Whitmore 1970; Weiland, Pless & Roghmann 1992). Incidence rates of the most common of chronic conditions are shown in Table 1.1, taken from a survey by Gortmaker (1985). This heterogeneous listing includes conditions which vary widely in terms of specific limitations, but they share one common feature. *All cannot be cured.* Modern medicine can, often very effectively, control pain, reduce the intensity of symptoms and limit the likelihood of long term complications, *but it cannot offer a cure.* Thus, children face a life-time of hospital appointments, diagnostic procedures and painful treatments. Every individual member of the child's family; parents, siblings, grandparents, uncles and aunts, will be touched and changed because of such a cruel and unexpected diagnosis. This book is about how these experiences with disease shape and influence children's development and relationships within the family.

Dimensions and characteristics of chronic diseases

Chronic diseases are characterised by their long duration and the fact that they cannot be cured. In other respects, they vary greatly. For a start, diseases vary in *aetiology*. Cystic fibrosis, spina bifida, cerebral palsy, phenylketonuria, are diagnosed before, at or soon after birth. Other conditions can occur at any time during childhood, although 'peak' incidences of certain diseases can occur within specific chronological ages (see Table 1.1). Diseases vary in *stability and predictability*. Children with arthritis, for example, generally have relatively stable health. This enables the child and parents to make plans for the future, since changes in health status (for better or worse) are unlikely to be sudden or dramatic. Other conditions are far from predictable. Asthma, epilepsy, diabetes, are all characterised by sudden and unexpected attacks. Being unable to predict the course of the disease raises practical and emotional problems for many families. Cancer, too is unpredictable. Children may very suddenly become ill, allowing families little time to reorganise their lives. Throughout treatment, parents need to keep a vigilant eye on their children, as reduced immunity which is a consequence of treatment leaves them vulnerable to many infections. While families are aware of the risks involved, illness episodes can be quite unexpected. Recurrences of the cancer can also occur without warning, and families live in fear of them. Some diseases, including muscular dystrophy, and to a lesser extent, cystic fibrosis, are *degenerative*. For these children and their families, the future is indeed unpredictable, and many live in hope of a miracle cure.

Diseases also vary in degree to which they represent an immediate *threat to life*. Modern medicine has changed the nature of potentially life-threatening conditions, such as cancer, diabetes, and cystic fibrosis. While all these could prove fatal if untreated, the discovery of new drugs and use of radiation and surgery has changed the nature of these diseases from life-threatening to chronic. Without treatment, most cancers would be associated with a rapid decline in health and early death. Dramatic improvements in survival have been attributed to the use of combinations of anti-cancer drugs, and refinements in irradiation and surgical procedures. Life expectancy for children with diabetes is now virtually the same as for the rest of the population. Antibiotics have done much to improve survival in cystic fibrosis. Conditions such as asthma more rarely result in premature death, but modern treatments have been very successful in controlling the frequency and intensity of attacks in all but the most severe of cases.

Diseases also vary in the extent to which prescribed treatments impose on and interrupt daily routines; particularly, they vary in *complexity and demandingness*. Many children with asthma may only need to take medication when an attack feels imminent; others may require more complex and rigorous medications frequently. Treatment for cancer is aggressive and painful, but generally conducted in hospital. Parents themselves have limited responsibilities for the medical care of their child. In other cases, parents (and the children if they are old enough) are encouraged to become as self-sufficient as possible. Management of diabetes, for example, requires daily monitoring of blood sugar levels, injections of insulin, and careful attention to diet. Similarly, management of cystic fibrosis requires patients and their families to be responsible for their own diets, physiotherapy and medication. Thus, diseases vary in the extent to which they require home or hospital based treatments. Home based treatments can be time-consuming and create friction between parent and child. Parents normally are concerned to make their children feel well and comfortable. Where they are also responsible for administering treatment regimens they may add to their child's discomfort, at least in the short term. In requiring parents to be responsible for frequent and unpleasant treatments, there is a risk of jeopardizing the natural trust between child and parent, and aggravating parent-child conflict.

Diseases differ in terms of the *restrictions* they place on the child's life. Well controlled asthma or epilepsy, for example, should present few (if any) practical restrictions, and for many purposes, children with these conditions should lead normal lives. Indeed, people who know the child only slightly may be unaware of the diagnosis. In other conditions, restrictions may result from limited cognitive abilities. Drugs used to control asthma and epilepsy, and treatments used in the control of leukemia, have all been associated with cognitive impairments in some children. Children with other conditions, such as muscular dystrophy or cerebral palsy, may experience motor restrictions as a direct consequence of the disease. Motor activity is limited by wasted muscle or organic brain damage.

Most chronic diseases, however, are not associated with damage of this kind. In these cases, restrictions can still be experienced, but less directly, and often through parental anxiety or lack of knowledge. For example, Markova, MacDonald and Forbes (1980) found that parents of boys with haemophilia limited their children's play and experience with potentially dangerous objects (such as knives) in an attempt to control the environment and reduce the possibility of accidents and bleeding episodes. Such limited experiences meant that, when they had to use knives or scissors, the boys were more likely to hurt themselves than healthy boys who had learned appropriate ways to handle sharp implements.

Children can also experience *social restrictions*. Again, the restrictions can be a direct consequence of the disease; children may feel tired or ill so that they are less likely to enjoy activities outside regular school hours, or attend school less regularly than others. The restrictions can also operate indirectly. Parents may limit the child's freedom to go out alone or discourage certain activities which they perceive to be associated with the potential for injury or accidents. Thus, boys may be discouraged from joining the local football club, just in case accidents happened.

The distinction between disease, disability and handicap

These terms are often used interchangeably, although disease generally refers to the biological basis of the condition, and disability or handicap to the behavioural consequences.

The classification schema adopted by the World Health Organization (1980) for the definitions of disabilities, impairments and handicaps makes the following distinctions. Impairments relate to any loss or abnormality of psychological, physiological or anatomical structure or function. Disabilities may be defined as the 'consequence of an impairment'. Handicaps more generally refer to the 'social disadvantage of a disability' and may limit or prevent the fulfillment of normal roles (Liptak 1987). Thus, they represent the consequences of disability or handicap and may have psychosocial and economic repercussions for the individual and society. Thus, as a result of a tumor in the leg, a child may undergo surgery for an amputation. The resulting disability is clearly visible in the loss of the leg, but the meaning of this handicap is socially and culturally determined. The child may become alienated from healthy peers and progressively isolated, or successfully be integrated with others in similar positions. A child who was active physically may participate in wheelchair athletics or find new sports which can be enjoyed despite the disability.

Themes of the book

One disease or several?

This book is concerned with how children and their families cope with chronic disease. Yet, given the extent and diversity of chronic conditions, we should ask how justified we are in considering them all together under one heading. At least two alternative theoretical perspectives can be identified. One reflects the prevailing medical point of view; all diseases are different and have specific implications for treatment. These include potential restrictions and the extent to which they disrupt family life or the child's potential to gain independence and autonomy. This view is associated with a perspective that looks at the consequences of a specific disease for child and family functioning. Many specialist journals and books (for example *Journal of Asthma; Diabetic Medicine; Epilepsia*) reflect this approach. It is characterised by research which attempts to describe idiosyncratic consequences of the condition and the development of measures suitable only for the specific population of individuals suffering from one disease. Thus, there are scales to measure 'quality of life' or adjustment in children and adolescents with diabetes (Challen *et al.* 1988; Jacobson *et al.* 1988) or cancer (Boggs, Graham-Pole & Miller 1991); or to measure self-efficacy in diabetes (Grossman, Brink & Hauser 1987) and asthma (Schlosser & Havermans 1992). The disadvantage of this approach is that it is not clear how far any difficulties identified are the result of specific characteristics or limitations of the disease, and how far they can be attributable to dimensions which cut across other diseases.

The alternative perspective stresses that many similarities hold across different conditions. According to this 'noncategorical' approach (Pless & Pinkerton 1975; Stein & Jessop 1982; Varni & Wallander 1988), families with a child with a chronic disease are confronted by a series of stressful situations. These include major life stresses (hospitalization, depletion of financial resources) and daily hassles (having to help dress the child or make special arrangements for transportation) over and above the stresses which confront all families on a routine basis. Proponents of this approach argue that the similarities in these demands, coupled with the infrequency at which specific chronic diseases occur in the population, make it more expedient to consider them within an overall framework. Certainly, it may often be more beneficial to make recommendations for children with chronic disease generally, rather than for any single disease alone. For example, we may wish to suggest that children with cancer need remedial education in school. Yet education authorities may be reluctant to initiate special services for such a small group of children. Arguments about why special educational provision should be made may seem stronger by considering all children with any chronic disease, since special provision can surely be justified for a group which constitutes 10 per cent or more of the school population.

What is perhaps important is not the *label* attached to the disease, but the extent to which the disease and treatments disrupt the family's ability to maintain everyday activities. For example, there is little point in considering all children with cancer under one heading. Some cancers (e.g. leukemia) are associated with relatively good prognosis, while treatment of other cancers (e.g. brain tumours) has progressed more slowly and the prognosis is far less easy to predict. On the surface, cancer and cystic fibrosis are very different; cancer has no known cause, but cystic fibrosis is inherited; cancer requires almost no patient responsibility for self-care, whereas cystic fibrosis requires a great deal. But both are life-threatening. In both, children are particularly vulnerable to childhood infections, either through lowered immunity as a result of chemotherapy, or through a general susceptibility to infection. Both therefore require families to explain to schools and neighbours that they must be told of outbreaks of chicken-pox or measles. Both require regular trips to hospital and frequent diagnostic tests. Both require a great deal of vigilance from parents and sensitivity to changes in the child's physical health and emotional well-being. This, and other prac-

tical demands may mean that there is more similarity between conditions as experienced by families than ever realised by medical personnel.

The need for a developmental framework

Regardless of the theoretical perspective adopted, there is a need for a
developmental approach in assessing the impact of chronic disease on
children and their families. I would define 'developmental' in the broad-
est of terms. The relatively rapid physical, cognitive and emotional
changes that take place during childhood create many difficulties compared with comparable work concerned with the impact of physical
disease on adults. Perhaps the most remarkable finding in all the literature is the extent to which children with chronic disease grow physically
and mentally in ways which are largely indistinguishable from the rest
of the population. Yet this development is in itself a problem for researchers; assessment must always be made against a background of
change and non-predictability. How can we ever say how chronic disease has affected a child, when we can never know what other variables
would have affected development in the absence of disease? There are,
in any case, different practical and emotional consequences of disease
depending on whether the sick child is two years old, five years old, or
adolescent. Issues of communication and explanations of the disease
and treatment necessarily vary with the child's cognitive ability.

These points are most explicitly made by Kazak (1989), who stresses
that care-taking demands can be viewed as normal if shared with
mothers of children of a particular age, whether or not the children have
a chronic disease. Care-taking demands become more problematic if the
child continues to need help beyond the normal period. A two-year-old
with a motor disease may need much help with physical activities and
have to be carried a great deal, but since all two-year-olds require this
kind of help families may not perceive it to be too problematic. The same
situation is much more difficult for the family of an older child. In any
case it is exhausting to carry a bigger child around all the time. Perhaps
more importantly, such behaviour is inappropriate and at variance with
the way in which other families behave towards their children. The need
to continue to provide this kind of help to the child beyond the normal
period is a constant reminder of the child's disease, and also creates a
divide between the family of the sick child and those of contemporaries.

'Caring for an infant with a motor delay is different from parenting
an adolescent who is confined to a wheel-chair. The additions of
other children to the family, divorces, deaths of grandparents, financial problems, relocations, and inclusions of other non-blood kin in
the family system are all 'normal' events families experience that
will affect the way in which the child's illness is perceived and
handled over time' (Kazak 1989, p.26).

In the pursuit of 'representative' samples, the methodology adopted in psychological work tends to mimic work in experimental psychology as far as possible. This results in attempts to coerce all children treated in a clinic into research programmes. At the extremes, this may mean that families with children ranging in age from pre-school to adolescence are asked the same questions about their own, and the children's response to the disease. Similarly, assumptions are made that adjustment difficulties or coping resources are purely a function of the disease, and independent of developmental processes. It has only recently begun to be acknowledged that children's appraisal of their situation, their resources to deal with the disease and its consequences, and their capacity to utilize external resources changes throughout childhood. By categorising children primarily by disease, much research has failed to consider the developmental issues of relevance in this context. More appropriate methodologies have as their focus a group of children within a narrow age-range, in order to facilitate the measurement of tasks appropriate to normal functioning (e.g. Quittner 1992).

Although 'development' most usually refers to the child, families also undergo systematic change. Issues confronting families of preschool children are not the same as those confronting families of adolescents. The fashion, until recently, for developmental psychology to focus on individuals under 16 years or so also means that some developmental concerns of parents have been overlooked. Developmental issues facing young parents (finding a house, establishing oneself at work) differ from those of middle-aged parents (caring for their own elderly relatives, acknowledging that they are no longer in line for promotion).

In addition, diseases themselves follow a developmental course. On diagnosis, families must deal with their shock and disbelief about what has happened, assimilate vast amounts of illness information and learn how to care for their child. These challenges change during the course of treatment. Families must learn how to integrate treatment demands with everyday work and social activities, keep hopeful, and define limits to the child's behaviour which take into account the child's need to attain independence, while balancing any constraints imposed by the disease. The bereaved family has to put the meaning of the child's life into some perspective and learn to live with the knowledge of the child's death. The dilemma is between keeping the memory of the child alive while at the same time creating an environment in which the living can achieve some fulfilment.

Theories of child development

Although it is increasingly acknowledged that the impact of chronic disease will vary depending on the child's developmental level, very little work has attempted to describe these differences empirically. There are a number of methodological reasons for this. Some diseases tend to be diagnosed within defined age-groups, precluding the possibility that impact can be assessed across childhood more generally. The incidence of leukemia, for example, peaks among 4-year-old children (Siegel 1980). Similarly, peaks in occurrence of diabetes have been noted in 5–6- and 11–13-year-old children (Drash 1979). In epilepsy, the most common ages of onset are five and seven years (Sands 1982).

Even where the incidence of a disease occurs more evenly throughout childhood, difficulties arise over the selection of measures that are appropriate across a wide age-range. This results from the practice of drawing samples from defined clinic populations. Given the relative rareness of any individual chronic condition, in order to collect a respectable sample size it is necessary to include children across a broad age-range. Consequently, the number of testing instruments available is limited, and those that are available are invariably insufficiently sensitive to detect the degree of change to be expected. The procedure raises difficulties even in the selection of intelligence tests, which invariably target a narrower age-range than is used in practice. The result is that insufficiently sensitive tests are used, or that children are required to complete measures which have been standardized on quite different populations.

Reasonable sample sizes can only be obtained therefore, by extensive collaboration between different treatment centres. Such studies are difficult to organise, and raise practical problems in terms of involving large numbers of individuals across wide geographical areas. To date, extensive collaboration of this kind has largely been limited to work with children with rare cancers both in Europe and the United States. A recent collaboration of pediatricians in the US is now committed to collaborative research and this may facilitate multicentre work in the future (Nazarian, Maiman & Bocker 1989).

For all these reasons, our understanding of the impact of disease on children at different developmental levels is essentially theoretical, and based on hypotheses drawn from theories of normal child development. This theoretical approach is then substantiated as far as possible by related empirical work. The most common theoretical approach adopted is rooted in cognitive developmental psychology. Choice of this theoretical framework has led to certain predictions about the types of behaviour to be studied as well as determining the methods of data collection.

Cognitive approaches

Both Perrin and Gerrity (1984) and Cerreto (1986) draw extensively on the theoretical work of Erikson (1959; 1964) and Piaget (1929, 1952). These theoretical frameworks are based on the assumption that certain developmental tasks need to be attained within a given age range; attainment of these tasks is considered to be the hallmark of healthy growth and development. The assumption is that maturation and experience interact to enable the child to achieve particular tasks and proceed to the next developmental level. Physical, psychological and environmental processes may interfere with the normal sequence of attainments, and chronic illness is perceived to constitute one such potential threat.

INFANT AND TODDLER YEARS

Chronic illness is a challenge to normal cognitive, social, emotional and physical development during this period. Separations from parents for medical treatment may be expected to disrupt the development of trust and attachment. The sick infant is likely to be handled by numerous care-takers and subjected to painful and uncomfortable procedures. These experiences may well limit the establishment of a basic trust which is thought to be the cornerstone of infant development. Reduced opportunities to play, explore and develop a close relationship with the family constitute hazards to normal development in infancy.

Cognitively, the toddler begins to use imagery and memory and learns through conditioning and rote learning. The characteristic of this period is 'egocentrism', or inability to differentiate the self from others and the world. Thus, the toddler assumes that personal experiences are shared by others and is unable to appreciate alternative perspectives. Toddlers attempt to become increasingly self-reliant, and consequently may conflict with adults who are more skeptical about the virtues of toddler independence. The achievements of this period are impressive; toddlers learn to walk, talk and control bodily processes. They are great explorers and endlessly curious. Yet their relationships with others can be fraught; parents may appear to block or interfere with many of their activities, and social play with peers is poorly developed and often insular. Toddlers can pursue their own idiosyncratic games while surrounded by other toddlers doing the same. Tantrums and fights over toys are commonplace, and toddlers need to be encouraged to share and consider others.

Given the limited verbal ability, it is difficult to prepare infants for medical procedures. They can be cuddled to console or reassure them, but little else can be done to compensate for the invasiveness and threat of procedures. Parents and staff can only hope that the infant will quickly forget the trauma.

PRESCHOOL AND EARLY SCHOOL YEARS

The process of attaining independence through exploration and discovery continues during the preschool period. Fine motor skills and general muscle control accelerates. Children begin to learn about cultural norms and expectations, about sex roles and the distinction between right and wrong. Children become more affectionate, adept at imitation, but still find it difficult to empathise with others in general situations. Some children experience frequent nightmares and phobias, and the fear of losing a part of their body.

The child's enjoyment of, and willingness to draw has been capitalised on as a means of acquiring data about the child's awareness of the body and how it works. In the conventional paradigm, children are given outline drawings of a body and asked to 'draw what it looks like inside' (Crider 1981). Preschool children think that the inside of their bodies is made up of blood, bones and food. Some also report that there is a heart 'for loving'. Beliefs about the cause of illness have variously been attributed to punishment for transgressions (Langford 1948) or magic (Bibace & Walsh 1981). It is easy to see how children with diabetes may see that treatments which involve limiting sweet foods and chocolate are a direct result of eating too many sweets in the past. Death is seen as a reversible process, and children deny their own mortality.

Children's understanding of illness and treatment is often regarded as rather 'cute'. They may explain very seriously that they fell over and hurt themselves, but 'mummy gave me a bag of crisps and made it better'. The child's limited linguistic skills (and our hesitation to develop alternative methods of eliciting the child's knowledge) may mean that we have seriously underestimated the child's understanding. A different picture emerges when alternative methodologies are adopted. Kendrick et al. (1986) based their study on observations of childrens' behaviour and interactions on the hospital ward. Children between two and three years of age with cancer picked up much more information about their condition than would have been expected. Much of this information was acquired through conversations and explanations given by other (more experienced) children.

One problem for cognitive theories is that although many children, with little or no experience of hospitals and illness, hold naive or cute ideas about its cause or implications, others can show considerable sophistication. A three-year-old girl with leukemia, for example, was able to give a relatively accurate and detailed account of the disease.

'I got leukemia. It just happens. I full of bad blood. Blood is red cells which make new blood; white cells which fight infection, and plate-lets which stop you bleeding. Sometimes the platelets don't come and then you keep bleeding'.

'How do the doctors make you better?'

'The bad cells just come. The doctors take the bad blood out. Then they get an enormous syringe and put new blood in. You have bone-marrows and lumbar punctures, but it never hurts'.

The child is able to repeat a relatively accurate account of the structure of blood and function of different blood cells; far more sophisticated, in fact, than given by many older children (Eiser, Havermans & Casas, 1993). Where she is less accurate is in her belief that she is all bad blood, and that doctors can replace all of it with good blood. In fact, the aim of chemotherapy is to destroy progressively some of the 'bad blood', allowing the 'good blood' to establish itself and become dominant. She has difficulty with understanding that her body can simultaneously contain both good and bad blood, a concept which is hard to grasp even for some adults. The belief that 'it never hurts' reflects the fact that small children are anesthetized routinely before bone-marrows and lumbar punctures, procedures which are extremely painful but necessary in order to establish the balance between good and bad cells throughout treatment.

THE MIDDLE SCHOOL YEARS

According to Piaget (1952), the cognitive achievements of this period include the attainment of concepts of conservation and reversibility, and the ability to use logical operations. Children learn to generalize from specific to general situations and instances, and are increasingly able to control and regulate their own behaviour. School is an important and pervasive aspect of the child's life; according to Erikson (1959) the foundations of 'industry' are laid down. Children learn to read and through reading are able to acquire extensive information in other areas.

As children spend time in school and with peers, the influence of the family declines. Children need to develop relationships with other adults, as well as establish friendship groups. Gender differences be-come pronounced, especially in preferences for different play activities and relationships with peers.

Bibace and Walsh (1981) distinguish two phases in the child's under-standing of illness. During the earlier period, *contamination*, children perceive the cause of illness to be external to themselves, but acknow-ledge a specific link between the source (germs, dirt) and the effect on the body. During the later stages of this period, thinking about illness is characterized by *internalization*. The cause of illness is seen to be internal to the body, and some relationships are perceived between cause and cure. Even so, childrens' awareness of the workings of their own bodies is minimal. With age, children are able to name an increasing number of body parts (Eiser & Patterson 1983), but are still largely ignorant about the function of different body parts or how they work together.

The impact of chronic disease is as much social as physical; children's concerns centre on their relationships with other children as well as with the implications of treatment. The issue is how to minimise the impact of the disease, so that as few people as possible know about the diagnosis. Children may go to some lengths to achieve this. Where cancer chemotherapy results in loss of hair, children will wear wigs. Those with diabetes are careful to eat discretely before exercise, so as not to appear different from everyone else. Children with chronic diseases generally can push themselves to their limits; doing school sports when they are tired, or going to school on days when they feel ill, when 'healthy' children would expect to stay home. Often, though, they fail to achieve the anonymity they desire. Parents and teachers find it hard not to make some allowances for the illness. More especially, other children can create conflict by teasing and focussing on aspects of the illness which prove difficult to hide. Ignorance about the cause of diseases can fuel further stereotyping and scapegoating.

'The other children in school don't like Thomas because he's got leukemia. They think they will get it too' (8-year-old sister).

THE ADOLESCENT YEARS

Rapid physical growth creates dramatic changes in body image. Physical maturity can change the way adolescents see themselves, as well as their relationships with others. New expectations about appropriate behaviour go hand in hand with the physical developments. Issues of sexuality, of concern about the future, and career choice are important for adolescents. Rapid physiological changes are often accompanied by mood swings and adolescents may become very difficult to live with.

A new stage of thought, or formal operations, emerges, as adolescents are less dependent on objects and imagery as props for thinking, and are able to comprehend abstract or symbolic ideas. Learning takes on an additional function as knowledge is applied to specific contexts and towards career choice. Adolescents need to establish independence from the nuclear family, while retaining close ties. Elkind (1967) describes a new form of egocentrism whereby adolescents refuse to acknowledge their own vulnerability, and are more prepared to take risks than at any other time in their lives.

Experience and formal biology teaching combine to fashion the adolescent's beliefs about illness and physiological functioning of the body so that increasingly accurate scientific and medical accounts are achieved. Adolescents understand that illness can occur through the break-down of a specific body part. Thus, adolescents with diabetes have no difficulty in ascribing the cause of the disease to the malfunctioning of the pancreas. They also recognise the individual's role in precipitating illness episodes, as well as the importance of self-care in treatment. At the most sophisticated level of functioning, adolescents understand the *psychophysiological* basis of illness, in which psychological determinants of illness causation and cure are called into play. Adolescents understand how mental states affect the body; they may, for example, perceive that illness can be precipitated by stressful events and conversely that recovery can be hampered by continuing stress levels.

Thus, adolescents themselves may feel that successful treatment requires more than simply 'doing what the doctor says'. Adolescents with cancer may look to alternative medicine to help them attain some personal control of their disease. They understand that their anger about the diagnosis may itself limit the possibility of cure, and seek out individuals or therapies which are reputed to promote adjustment and Through alternative medicine, they hope to find some inner peace, and ultimately control the spread of cancer cells.

The special case of diabetes

A related analysis, specific to the impact of diabetes, has been proposed by Cerreto and Travis (1984) and Anderson (1990). Diabetes is the most common endocrine disorder in children, resulting from insufficient insulin production by the pancreas. Insulin is vital for energy utilization; onset of the disorder is therefore indicated by extreme tiredness, and weight loss despite above normal eating and drinking. Treatment involves daily blood tests to monitor blood sugar levels (hemoglobin) and injections of insulin to mirror as far as possible normal production. The process is complicated, however, given the shifts in insulin requirements resulting from food intake, exercise, stress or illness. Diabetes requires careful monitoring of blood- sugar levels and dietary restrictions. The essence of treatment for diabetes is self-care; patients and families are encouraged to be responsible themselves for much of the necessary treatment. While this falls heavily on families initially, older children must increasingly assume responsibility for their own health care.

More than many other conditions, diabetes requires families to develop ways of balancing the growing child's needs for independence and autonomy with the family support and involvement necessary for self-care and successful implementation of treatment. establishes the acceptance. The ways in which the child responds to treatment restrictions and establishes the means to deal with them is described by Cerreto and Travis (1984) and Anderson (1990) using the same theoretical schema as described above:

INFANT AND TODDLER YEARS

Specific management problems facing parents with a child under three years old include: monitoring blood sugar control; establishing regular meal-times regardless of whether or not the child is hungry; helping the child to accept the need for insulin injections (even though the child does not feel ill and does not feel any different after the injection); and managing conflicts with other siblings (who are invariably also very young and therefore unable to understand the reasons for the extra attention that appears to be made of the child with diabetes), (Leaverton 1979). During this period, there is no question but that parents are exclusively responsible for the child's treatment. Their difficulties centre on the impossibility of explaining the need for treatment to the child in any comprehensible form, and the fact that much treatment, particularly in its requirement for frequent and regular meal-times, is so much at odds with a toddler's preferred eating habits.

PRE-SCHOOL AND EARLY SCHOOL YEARS

During this period, the family faces some new challenges as it becomes necessary to manage diabetes outside the home setting. For many parents, school entry is associated with the need to explain diabetes to people outside the nuclear family and close friends. Parents must accept that they are no longer responsible for the child during the school day, and trust teachers to act appropriately if the child shows signs of illness at school. For the first time, parents may need to act as 'diabetes educators' in order to ensure that the school understands the nature of the disease and the practical steps to be taken if the child shows signs of hyper- (too much blood sugar) or hypo-glycemia (too little blood sugar).

School attendance also enables the child with diabetes to mix socially with other children, perhaps heightening their awareness of disease-related restrictions. Lack of cooperation with the diet is particularly acute in this period, (Bregani *et al.* 1979) as children may demand to have sweets and junk foods with their friends. Invitations to birthday parties require that parents make more explanations to strangers. Children with diabetes may be prevented from going to parties, or mothers may go to great lengths to provide suitable foods which are specially sent from home (Eiser, Patterson & Town 1985).

THE MIDDLE SCHOOL YEARS

The characteristic of this period is the child's move toward independence and involvement in self-care. The way in which families resolve the dilemmas created by the child's need for independence with their attempts to teach and supervise is likely to have an almost immediate effect on metabolic control, as well as influencing much longer-term attitudes to treatment and adherence. Problems can arise where families fail to communicate accurately about who is responsible for various aspects of treatment. Allen et al. (1983) identified diet management as a particular source of conflict, and it is in this area that most direct conflict with other family members was also likely. Many parents reported adopting a variety of techniques, such as forestalling sibling rivalry over snacks, to lessen family conflict. However, it is in relation to responsibility for insulin injections that conflicts between parents and the child with diabetes most frequently occur. Transference of responsibility may be a major hurdle, and many parents expressed relief when they were no longer required to administer injections to their child.

Bregani et al. (1979) also identified this period as one in which children become more acutely aware of the ways in which they differed from healthy peers, with some negative consequences for the child in terms of loss of self-esteem and feelings of inadequacy. In the study reported by Allen et al. (1983), peer conflict created special obstacles to adherence to dietary advice. The need for frequent meals and snacks, and restriction of junk foods and sweets, can separate the child with diabetes from others.

THE ADOLESCENT YEARS

The adolescent needs to become virtually self-sufficient in terms of implementing self-care activities. The adolescent needs to become personally responsible for all aspects of treatment, while families withdraw their involvement to little more than occasional surveillance (Cerreto & Travis 1984). Potential conflicts can remain from earlier periods over who exactly is responsible for treatment. Parents, especially mothers, frequently express concern that the adolescent is less conscientious about these responsibilities than is necessary. As is true for all parent–child relationships, conflicts can become particularly intense. Issues of independence and autonomy characterize most parent–child conflicts, but can be aggravated where parents perceive that the child's behaviour or failure to implement treatment appropriately can be life-threatening.

As the influence of the family decreases, the peer-group becomes more important. Treatments can be compromised so that the adolescent does not lose face with others. Dilemmas also occur as the adolescent is tempted to experiment with alcohol or drugs, and the impact on insulin requirements is increasingly challenged. Adolescents with diabetes need to establish support groups outside the family who are sympathetic to, and aware of, the potential role that may be sometimes necessary in helping the young adult with diabetes.

Issues of sexuality, obtaining life insurance and making career choices become paramount. With the move to independent living, adolescents and young adults find that their treatments need to be fitted in with their new life-styles and those of their partners. Balancing the needs of the treatment with demands of others is aggravated by the birth of children.

'The baby cries a lot and I forget about my insulin. I always feed her before we eat ourselves. It's so busy with the baby. I sit down to eat and realise I've forgotten to take my insulin. I have to try to remember my injection as I put the potatoes on' (New mother with long-standing diabetes).

Criticisms of the cognitive approach

General criticisms of the cognitive approach have been extensive (e.g. Gellman & Baillargeon 1983). Objections have centred on the difficulties in explaining how children proceed from one developmental stage to the next, and why understanding of various concepts can occur simultaneously across different stages. Objections have also been raised about the focus on cognitive processes without regard for the social and cultural context within which change occurs (Nelson 1986). The cognitive approach is also increasingly recognized as inadequate to account for how children perceive their illness and understand its causes and limitations. Examples, such as the three-year old with her quite impressive account of leukemia, abound, and challenge the idea that children's understanding of their own illness is limited by cognitive operations. The essence of much criticism is that illness occurs in a social context, and theories which do not take this into account are necessarily inadequate (Nelson 1986; Eiser 1989; Hergenrather & Rabinowitz 1991).

Social-ecology theory

A second approach stresses the role of the social context in determining children's response to disease and treatment. The social context can include the child's immediate and extended family, as well as larger societal groups, such as school, neighbourhood and the hospital. Social ecology theory emphasises the relationship between the developing child and the social contexts in which interactions occur. The assumption is that the child is at the centre of a series of concentric rings, with the nested circles representing larger environments with which the child must interact (Bronfenbrenner 1979).

The innermost ring represents the family, or 'microsystem'. This is followed by the 'mesosystem' or smaller settings, such as school or hospital where the child interacts. Third, the 'exosystem', includes settings which do not include the child directly but influence the child through other family members. Included in this category would be parents' work- colleagues or friends, as well as friends and teachers of siblings. Thus, consideration of the social context in which children learn to cope with chronic disease must include attention to the structure, function and resources of each of the above three systems (Kazak 1992).

Table 1.1 Incidence and survival data for childhood chronic disease; adapted from Gortmaker (1985)

Disease	Age of onset 1000 live births	Incidence per estimates	Survival
Cystic fibrosis	variable, usually in the 1st year	0.50	70% to 21 years
Spina bifida	birth	1.00	45% to 4–8 years
Leukemia	any time	0.03	60% survival
Congenital heart disease	usually in the 1st year	8.00	52% to 15 years
Asthma	variable	10.0	similar to normal
Sickle cell disease	latter part of first year	0.36	95% to 20
Kidney disease	variable	2.00	similar to normal
Diabetes	peak at 12 years	0.40	95% to 20
Muscular dystrophy	after 3 years	0.14	25% to 20
Hemophilia	90% by 3–4 years	0.13	normal to 20 years
Cleft plate	birth	0.40	normal

To date his theory has generated less empirical work that the cognitive approach.

Social ecological approaches stress the reciprocal nature of human relationships. The question is not simply 'how does chronic disease affect this child?' The child is seen to be active in determining or shaping the response of others, and, in turn, significant others have a part to play in shaping the behaviour of the child. The approach stresses the importance of natural transitions and changes which occur in childhood; thus, it is not a static model. Instead, it is recognised that growth and change characterise childhood and relationships within families. Understanding the impact of chronic disease can only be assessed within a framework in which these changes can be assimilated.

CHAPTER 2

Chronic Disease in Infancy

The birth of a new baby is usually a very happy occasion and, certainly for many parents, the period immediately following the birth is generally perceived very positively. Parents may experience considerable relief that the birth is over, that there were no complications, and that the baby is healthy. Hospital staff are available to help with the practical side of care, and play an important role in teaching new parents how to handle their tiny, very slippery baby! Friends and relatives, too, are often keen to visit and offer their congratulations, and invariably confirm parents' views that the child is indeed extremely beautiful. At this time, parents may be blissfully unaware of how very demanding a healthy baby can be, especially where little practical help is available from professionals or family. Inexperience with small babies and lack of confidence in parenting roles can prove difficult for all new parents; does the baby eat enough, sleep enough, grow enough? The questions are multiplied for parents with a sick baby.

In many cases, there are no indications prior to the birth that anything is wrong. Parents' expectations for a normal healthy baby are suddenly violated, and they generally have no time in which to prepare themselves for the emotional crisis with which they are faced.

The intensive care unit
Both mothers and fathers report making many changes in their lifestyles prior to the birth of the child, and for this reason can feel particularly distressed and victimized when denied a normal birth and healthy baby (Affleck, Tennen & Rowe 1991). Both parents are likely to experience considerable distress in these circumstances, and these stresses are especially pronounced where the baby is born prematurely or seriously ill. Parents identify the intensive care environment itself as a source of much distress. It is highly technological and artificial, with unbelievably small babies attached to unbelievably large pieces of machinery. Parents are uncomfortable in this environment, and frightened to touch the child or upset the machinery. It can be very hot; staff are very busy, and the 'life-and-death' atmosphere that pervades is contagious and unnerving.

At the same time, parents are often required to make complex treatment decisions with far-reaching implications. The infant may be subject
to painful procedures, and parents often feel quite powerless, with no
clearly defined role to perform in caring for their child. Under these
circumstances, tensions can escalate, as parents and staff disagree about
treatments. Parents also identify difficulties with other relatives, who
may feel critical of the hospital care, or hold parents partially responsible
for the crisis. Added to the immediate stresses, parents may harbour real
anxieties about the implications for the child's future (Pederson *et al.*
1988; Affleck *et al.* 1986).

Mothers' responses
Mothers of premature and sick infants are more distressed immediately
after the birth and several months later than are mothers of healthy
infants (Trause & Kramer 1983). Mothers of premature infants perceive
their babies to be more fragile, weaker and more likely to die (DiVitto &
Goldberg 1979; Plunkett, Meisles & Stiefel 1986), and they feel that the
child is more likely to contract a life-threatening condition than healthy
infants (Briggs 1985). Throughout childhood, mothers of premature
infants continue to be more concerned than mothers of healthy children
about the physical health, strength and susceptibility to illness of their
children (Perrin, West & Culley 1989).

Fathers' responses
As is discussed more fully in Chapter 6, fathers of chronically sick
children are usually assigned a supportive role. It is generally mothers
who have most interaction with hospital staff, spend time in hospital
with the child and more openly express anxiety and concerns about the
future. Affleck, Tennen and Rowe (1990) acknowledge that the fathers
in their study were invariably assigned (or assigned themselves) to
supporting roles, but stress the potential benefits of mutual supportive
processes.

This general impression is confirmed by Davis (Davis & May 1991)
in describing his personal experience at the birth of an ill baby. He
suggests that the attitudes and advice given by medical staff can legiti-
mize the father's role in terms of support rather than encouraging a more
central role in care. Staff attitudes may be particularly critical at this time,
in that they may be influential in determining a pattern of care between
parents that characterizes their relationships with the child throughout
early life.

The period following hospital discharge
For these parents, it often seems that troubles are over when the baby is
out of intensive care and on the way home. In fact, they face many more

difficulties than do parents of healthy children. Parents may continue to feel a good deal of anxiety about their child, which may be aggravated by a continuing need to return with the child for medical check-ups. Infants often remain dependent on medical technology or daily treatments. In addition, such infants may look, behave and develop differently from healthy counterparts. For example, the cries of sick or premature babies are generally higher and sound more urgent than the cries of healthy babies (Lester & Zeskind 1979). Infants may well continue to experience feeding difficulties, make slow weight gain and be subject to frequent and recurring minor illnesses. Feeding difficulties are especially common in infants with congenital heart disease (Gillon 1972; Gudersmith 1975). Mothers also reported difficulties in anticipating and recognising the needs of the baby as well as in establishing early social interactions (Pinelli 1981; Gudersmith 1975). Parents themselves rapidly become exhausted by broken nights and the need for constant vigilance. Perceptions of the infant's vulnerability may result in parents feeling unable to leave the infant with anyone else. At the same time, the infant's real need for specialized care may genuinely lead to a limited number of potentially appropriate baby-sitters. Difficulties and conflicts with relations that began following the birth may well continue once the child is home, especially where continued slow development and progress is made.

Conditions diagnosed in infancy

As medical care has advanced, the health of the majority of babies has also improved. There remain however, a number of more serious and threatening conditions that are resistant to currently known treatments. Within these categories are congenital conditions such as cystic fibrosis, Tay-Sachs disease, phenylketonuria, haemophilia, epidermolysis bullosa (a severe and incapacitating condition which causes blistering of the skin), some heart conditions, and most recently AIDS. All are usually diagnosed within a few days (for example PKU) or months (for example cystic fibrosis) of birth.

Although it is not intended to discuss the details of these conditions and their treatment exhaustively, some analysis of the implications of diseases which are diagnosed during infancy is necessary in order to appreciate the impact on families. One of the most common potentially fatal conditions diagnosed during infancy is cystic fibrosis. This condition is genetically determined of autosomal recessive origin, and occurs where both parents are heterozygous carriers. In these cases, a couple have a one in four chance of an affected child.

The diagnosis of cystic fibrosis

Cystic fibrosis is caused by a defective pair of genes on chromosome number 7, and occurs only where both parents transmit the defective gene. Neither parent shows any symptoms themselves. The recessive nature of the disease requires the presence of both genes for manifestation. Thus, it is estimated that 1 in every 20 or 30 individuals are unknowing carriers of the recessive gene.

The disease itself is characterized by widespread dysfunction of the exocrine glands and is associated with many complications. Cystic fibrosis affects many parts of the body, including the lungs, liver and pancreas. It occurs in approximately 1 in every 2000 births. About 5 percent of patients also develop diabetes.

Treatment is palliative and involves efforts to minimize the complications of the disease, rather than the symptoms. Therapy involves control of diet, especially with regard to intake of enzymes and vitamins, administration of antibiotics, physiotherapy, and inhalation therapy. Children with cystic fibrosis almost always have some digestive problems, due to pancreatic deficiency. Although often ravenously hungry, malabsorption of food can result in undernourishment and poor growth. Administration of pancreatic enzymes before meals and/or a high protein, low fat diet is generally prescribed. These food supplements are advised throughout the life of the child. In addition to the dietary demands, families are responsible for daily physio- and drug-therapy. As soon as possible after diagnosis, postural drainage is necessary to clear up mucous from the lungs as aid to breathing and to slow down the course of infection. Inhalation therapy to break up and loosen mucous is also advised. As the child gets older, breathing exercises are taught to avoid overdevelopment of the chest.

Although, with appropriate therapy, infants and young children may be relatively well, the disease is progressive, and patients face a limited lifespan. Before the discovery of antibiotics, more than half of infants with cystic fibrosis died before two years of age, and more than three-quarters before the age of ten years (Schwachman & Kulczcki 1985). Current projections are more optimistic. Nevertheless, the practical and emotional stakes in caring for a child with cystic fibrosis remain extremely high, but better summarized by a father than any published statistics:

'It took a lot of pressure to get anyone to listen seriously to my wife and myself that anything was wrong. Martha was eventually diagnosed at two years after a year or so of constantly telling GPs, health visitors, etc, that things were wrong. At diagnosis in hospital, the consultants were astonishingly frank, stressing that (1) a handicapped child means a handicapped family; (2) what is worse than a handicapped child is a spoilt handicapped child; (3) quality, not quantity, of life, is what we should seek; (4) the life-threatening implications of cystic fibrosis were spelt out in no uncertain terms. The responsibility for treatment was placed firmly on our shoulders; this included two or three lots of percussion physiotherapy each day, (15 minutes a time), mixing and administering various medicines, administering a nebuliser machine; it was clearly up to us to keep our child free from infection. Martha is now responsible for all her own treatment (over 60 tablets each day, four injections, physiotherapy, food calculations and input). Although understanding that cystic fibrosis is an inherited condition caused by the meeting of recessive genes from the mother and father, we felt no guilt, though warned to expect it. We were far too busy trying to keep our daughter fit and well'.

Traditionally, diagnosis was difficult, and complaints about the time taken to reach satisfactory diagnoses are relatively common. Current screening practices are making delayed diagnoses less common; thus, one hopes, reducing parental uncertainty and improving prognosis for the child. It is important to begin therapy as soon as possible in order to delay onset of pulmonary complications, and ultimately extend life-expectancy.

It is, of course, unreasonable to expect infants and young children to cooperate with such invasive procedures, and consequently there are many opportunities for problems to develop between parents and their child. Not all parents manage ways of administering treatment which are acceptable to their children. The father of Martha considers this problem:

'During a lot of the daily treatment, Martha was in an immobile state. To pass the time, we used to read to her incessantly. As both parents were often involved in treatment, our other child quickly got the message that she too would have to listen to the stories.'

Psychological adjustment during infancy:
The development of attachment

In considering the impact of chronic disease during the infancy period, researchers have been concerned particularly with implications for parent-child attachment. According to attachment theory (Bowlby 1969; Bretherton & Waters 1985), a major achievement of the first year of life is the formation of a primary social attachment. The quality of this first relationship is assumed to be central to, and predictive of, much future development. Chronic disease is thought to jeopardize the normal attachment process by interfering with mothers' ability or desire to relate to the child in a way that would promote healthy social development.

First, parents may be separated from the child immediately following the birth, and sometimes for extended periods of time later, depending on the need for medical treatment. These separations are not inevitably associated with difficulties in parent-child relationships, but may aggravate other difficulties under certain circumstances.

Second, there is an emotional uncertainty about the child's future. Even if parents have been assured that the condition is not life-threatening, the infant is likely to be seen as very small, fragile, and potentially vulnerable. Parents may also see themselves as responsible for the child's condition, either because of a known hereditary component (for example, in haemophilia or cystic fibrosis), or because of something that they did during the pre-natal period. Mothers especially can blame themselves for eating particular foods, smoking, or working too hard during pregnancy (Affleck, Tennen & Rowe 1991).

Third, day-to-day care of the chronically sick infant can deviate substantially from that involved in caring for a healthy infant. In the least demanding situation, parents of an infant with cystic fibrosis are responsible only for administering enzymes with meals, but in many cases they must also give inhalation therapy and physiotherapy on a daily basis. These tasks are demanding in themselves, but also cut into time that might otherwise be used for play with the child, and recreation time for parents. The emotional relationship between sick or premature babies and their parents is potentially undermined in many ways; through increased anxiety and concern, through the demands of additional care-taking tasks and through a reduction in 'fun' time available together.

Much work suggests that interactions between mothers and their infants is affected by prematurity (Goldberg & DiVitto 1983), Down's syndrome (Jones 1980) and sensory handicaps (Goldberg 1982). These changes have variously been attributed to stress (Goldberg 1978), maladaptation (Field 1977), or seen to be appropriate given the special needs of the child (Goldberg & DiVitto 1983). Thus, mothers of premature infants are more active and directing in feeding and general interactions with their infants, and less likely to engage in any game-playing than mothers of healthy infants (Field et al. 1979). This may be appropriate given that the sick infant is sleepier and less likely to cooperate in the feeding process than a healthy baby.

Assessment of attachment

Attachment quality is typically assessed using the 'strange situation' (Ainsworth *et al.* 1978). In this procedure, child, mother and a friendly female stranger are brought into a playroom setting. Over a course of eight brief episodes, each of the adults departs and returns. On the basis of the child's behaviour, the mother-child dyad is categorized as:

1) secure. The child uses the parent as a secure base for exploration. Attachment behaviour (calling, searching, crying) is heightened when the parent leaves. On reunion, the child greets the parent positively, makes physical contact if distressed, settles, and returns to play.

2) Insecure/avoidant. The child is minimally distressed by separation, ignores or avoids the parent at reunion and seems to be preoccupied with exploration though very aware of the parent.

3) Insecure/resistant. The child explores minimally even with the parent present, is extremely distressed by departure, seeks contact on reunion but does not settle readily' (Goldberg *et al.* 1990, p.728).

Fischer-Fay *et al.* (1988) compared 23 infants with cystic fibrosis and their mothers with 23 mother-child pairs in whom there was no history of illness. There were no differences between the groups in terms of security of attachment, suggesting that the mother-child bond is relatively resilient, and that successful adaptation to the demands of the disease is possible. Within the cystic fibrosis group, however, it was found that insecurely attached infants had less than optimal physical growth. The insecurely attached infants were similar in weight for height compared with the healthy controls, but securely attached infants were 'chubbier' than normal controls. Securely and insecurely attached infants did not differ on medical criteria, such as lung-function, number of hospitalizations or degree of initial malabsorption. Of special significance, perhaps, was the fact that insecurely attached infants were diagnosed when younger compared with the securely attached infants.

There are, therefore, two unpredicted findings reported in this study. The first, that securely attached infants with cystic fibrosis were chubbier than normal infants; the second that infants who were diagnosed when younger were less securely attached than infants diagnosed later. This is contrary to most expectations, since it is generally assumed that early diagnosis is desirable. The finding has some implications for neonatal screening programmes, since it suggests that early diagnosis may create bonding difficulties for some mother-infant dyads. The study points to the advantages to be gained where mother and child are able to establish their relationship prior to the diagnosis of a life-threatening condition. These findings are provocative, and in need of replication on larger samples of infants, not least because they are relevant to very practical issues regarding the value of early screening programs and implications for counselling parents following the birth of a child with a congenital condition.

Goldberg *et al.* (1990) further investigated the potentially adverse effects of chronic disease on mother-infant relationships by comparing attachment in healthy infants with those suffering from cystic fibrosis or congenital heart disease. They predicted more secure attachment in the healthy infants than either of the sick groups, but also expected differences between the sick groups related to differences in treatments and prognoses. Cystic fibrosis is a progressive condition and involves much daily care by parents. In contrast, congenital heart disease includes a range of conditions, which differ in severity and prognosis. The majority are correctable by surgery, but often the long-term outcome is not clear during the infancy period. Parents may therefore experience much concern and anxiety, but be required to do less in the way of additional practical care than parents of infants with cystic fibrosis.

Attachment patterns did not differ across the three groups. The authors noted, however, that the pattern of responses was in the predicted direction, in that there was a higher proportion of securely attached infants in the healthy group. There were no apparent differences in qualitative aspects of attachment between those with cystic fibrosis or congenital heart disease. In cases of insecure attachment, infants tended to show *avoidant* patterns of behaviour, rather than *resistant*.

Infant's behaviour in the 'strange situation' has been considered important for current functioning and also for implications for future functioning. At least among normal infants, securely attached infants are more competent across a range of cognitive and social tasks than are insecurely attached infants (Ainsworth *et al.* 1978). Interest in attachment behaviour is therefore considerable, not only as an indicator of current mother-child behaviour, but also because security of attachment in infancy is often considered predictive of later functioning. At least among healthy infants, securely attached infants at one year were later found to be more sociable with peers (Park & Waters 1989), and unfamiliar adults. They are also reported to be better problem-solvers at school, more persistent and enthusiastic, and more socially competent (Block & Block 1980). Consistent with these findings is the notion that security of attachment is a reflection of 'quality mothering'. Securely attached infants have mothers who are more sensitive to the infant's needs. In contrast, there is accumulating evidence that avoidant infants have mothers who are insensitive, angry and intrusive, while ambivalent infants have mothers who can be characterised by their insensitivity, inept, and sometimes neglectful behaviour (Egeland & Sroufe 1981; Goldberg *et al.* 1986). Subsequent work has stressed the importance of the match between mother and infant characteristics (Belsky & Isabella 1988).

Goldberg *et al.* (1990) studied the growth of autonomy and independence at two years of age. Behaviour at two years was expected to relate to earlier attachment, the hypothesis being that securely attached infants would be more successful in negotiating independence and autonomy than insecurely attached infants, regardless of diagnostic grouping. Chronic disease was expected to affect adversely the mother-child relationship, with mothers being less supportive as well as exhibiting under- or over- controlling behaviour.

A puzzle-solving task developed by Matas, Arend and Sroufe (1978) was used. This consists of a series of graded puzzles; the initial ones being easily solved by the child alone. 'The way in which the adult provides support for the child at appropriate times and the way in which the child seeks and uses this assistance is rated' (Goldberg *et al.* 1990). According to Matas *et al.* (1978), children who were most securely attached in infancy interacted most successfully with their mothers to solve these tasks. This finding was confirmed for children in the healthy group; i.e., infants who were initially well-attached also appeared able to negotiate autonomy and independence more successfully at two years. The relationship was not supported for either of the groups of sick children.

The result that early attachment is not related to more harmonious mother-child relationships at two years among the chronically sick groups is consistent with other work suggesting few clear effects of attachment over time among children with a medical history. This is in contrast to results reported for healthy children. It seems that, for healthy children, the quality of early relationships are predictive of subsequent functioning under normal circumstances. Inversely, for normal children, poor initial attachments may be cause for concern. This is not necessarily so for chronically sick children. In these instances, diagnosis and treatment of the disease may well adversely affect mother-child attachment at least during the initial crisis. One implication of these data would be that such a compromise in early attachments is not necessarily irreversible; mothers and their children have some capacity for setting things right.

While such an interpretation has considerable appeal, it lacks any real empirical support. It is not clear from the data reported by Goldberg *et al.* (1990) how the child's current health status relates to dependence behaviour; i.e. whether those children who were first seen to be insecurely attached but who subsequently related well to their mothers in the puzzle-solving task were also those whose physical functioning had improved most effectively. It would also be important to know how mothers perceived their child's disease and prognosis. In the classic studies by Linde *et al.* (1966) children who were wrongly diagnosed to have heart conditions were subsequently found to be restricted compared with healthy children. Thus, mothers' beliefs about the child's health status determined activity level rather than the physical condition itself; there was no medical reason why these children should have been restricted in any way. The changes in interaction reported by Goldberg *et al.* (1990) between mothers and their sick infants may partly be accounted for by mothers' understanding of the nature of the condition and beliefs about restrictions. Future work needs to include some assessment of mothers' beliefs and attributions about children's growth and development as well as changes in physical status in order to understand the processes underlying any change in quality of mother-infant attachment.

In one of the most recent studies to be published by Goldberg and her colleagues (Goldberg *et al.* 1991) attachment behaviour was compared in 42 infants with congenital heart disease and 46 healthy infants. The results of this study parallel some of those reported earlier. More of the healthy infants were found to have secure attachments to their mothers than those with heart disease. Among the chronically ill group, security of attachment was not related to mothers' reports of their own stress or psychological well-being. As in the study reported by Fischer-Fay *et al.* (1988), there were suggestions that security of the mother-infant dyad was important to the health of the child. Securely attached infants showed more improvement in health over a one year period. Unlike the results reported previously, Goldberg *et al.* (1991) concluded that heart disease is a risk factor for mother-infant relationships, in that these infants were less likely to be securely attached than healthy infants.

Attempts have also been made to extend the use of the strange situation to assess attachment between fathers and their healthy infants. Cox, Owen, Henderson and Margand (1992) assessed parents' attitudes to the infant, their beliefs about their parenting role and the time spent with the infant. In addition, attachment was assessed on one occasion, between infants and their mothers, and on a second occasion between infants and their fathers. Infant-mother and infant-father attachment at one year could both be predicted from the nature of earlier interactions. Attachment was best predicted from a combination of variables including sensitivity, positive affect, reciprocal play, attitude to play, amount of vocalization, encouragement of achievement and physical affection. For fathers, attitudes to the infant were also important, with fathers who rated their role more highly having more securely attached infants.

Darke and Goldberg (unpublished manuscript) assessed father-infant interaction immediately following mother-infant interaction in the strange situation. As with mothers and their infants, security of attachment between fathers and their infants was less strong among those with an infant with heart disease than of healthy infants and their fathers or those with cystic fibrosis and their fathers. Darke and Goldberg also noted that many of these differences could be attributable to the behaviour of fathers rather than the infants. There is much evidence that fathers are less involved in direct care of infants with chronic conditions than mothers or fathers of healthy infants (see Chapter 5). The development of laboratory techniques such as this may play an important role in establishing how father-infant relationships are challenged and compromised by chronic disease.

The assessment of attachment behaviour is time-consuming, but few alternative methodologies have so far achieved wide acceptance. An exception is the Attachment Q-sort (Waters & Deane 1985). In this procedure, mothers or trained observers produce a Q-sort description of the child, which is then compared against a hypothetical 'most secure child' described by Waters and Deane (1985). This procedure, too, is quite cumbersome. Respondents are asked to complete a Q-sort according to a rectangular description (8 categories of 11 items, with the middle category receiving 12 items). Vaughn et al. (1992) noted that this procedure was unacceptable to a British sample, and a slightly modified and simplified format was necessary. Despite the methodological difficulties, work concerned with infant-mother attachment raises some important questions about what constitutes sensitive mothering, especially sensitive mothering of sick infants.

For normal infant mother pairs, Cox et al. (1992) operationalized sensitivity to include assessment of the extent to which parent-infant interaction was characterised by prompt and appropriate responses to the baby's signals. Related measures included the positiveness of parental affect; affective animation, ranging from flat emotionless expression to expressive face and sparkling eyes; the amount of reciprocal play; parents' attitude toward play; parents' activity level; and the parents' encouragement of achievement. The particular characteristics which define sensitive parenting of chronically sick infants need to be identified.

Psychological impact during the preschool period

Some authors have suggested that the second year of life is particularly difficult for families of sick and disabled children (Wasserman & Allen 1985). While cognitive, physical and social development in healthy children is rapid, slower progress is often observed in the chronically sick, and may be particularly acute in language and motor function. Mothers may increasingly become aware of differences between their own and healthy children (Jennings et al. 1985).

Parents of toddlers report more stress than parents of older children. Parents attempt to shape and mould their children's behaviour and conflicts are frequent. Two-year-olds are famous for temper tantrums and stubbornness, and in turn, attempt to fashion parental behaviour according to their own preferences. Parenting a two-year-old can sometimes seem to lurch from one showdown to another. Challenges are many; bedtimes, mealtimes, going shopping. Two-year-olds can be messy eaters at the best of times, as well as being fussy and unpredictable about what, or how much, they are prepared to eat. Parents' concern about children's eating and need to make adequate weight-gain can mean that many crises are precipitated over food. These are aggravated where parents have special concerns about the importance of good eating to combat the damaging effects of disease. For example, it is normally recommended that children with cystic fibrosis need a higher than normal calorific intake, in order to counter the malabsorption effects of the disease. Particularly when they are tired or ill, children may resist parents' efforts to coax food inside them, and food refusal and faddiness is common. The under-nourished child is irritable, and further refuses food; a cycle of poor eating and conflicts at mealtimes is the result.

Allen, Wasserman and Seidman (1990) investigated 37 three-year-old children with congenital abnormalities and their mothers with a control group of normal children and their mothers. The children suffered from a range of congenital syndromes, although almost half were diagnosed with cleft lip or palate or both. Mothers and their children were videotaped in free play or teaching situations together. Children were also videotaped in solitary play.

The results suggest fewer differences between children with congenital conditions and peers than might be expected. Children with congenital conditions were as cooperative as normal children in both the free play and teaching tasks, and significantly more cooperative in clearing up at the end of the activity! These children were less likely to make demands on their mothers during play and were as self-reliant as normal children during free play. Overall, there appeared to be little evidence that mothers of children with congenital conditions were more intrusive and negative in interactions with their children than healthy mother-child pairs. However, there were some signs of unusual behaviour. Mothers of the children with congenital conditions were twice as likely to give orders or distract their child in the teaching situation. They were also more likely to try to engage their children through nonverbal, rather than verbal interactions. Allen, Wasserman and Seidman (1990) concluded that the preschool period may be a time when few differences as a function of health status were apparent, although it was also noted that infants with congenital conditions were more passive and compliant. Future work needs to untangle whether this can be attributed to differences in parenting, or is a response to hospitalization, intrusions from treatment and separations from the normal family environment.

Most research seems to suggest that mother–child interactions during the infancy/toddler period are not grossly distorted by the occurrence of disease or congenital abnormalities. Yet there are also some consistent differences between these and healthy dyads. In particular, the children themselves seem relatively passive and nonresponsive, and mothers themselves appear less affectionate and involved. It would be easy to conclude that the disease or abnormality was directly responsible for the mother's behaviour. However, one might suggest that a number of other variables may also be involved. Infants with any medical condition are inevitably exposed to many medical interventions and may also experience repeated separations from parents as a result of hospitalization. In addition, many conditions that affect infants are associated with feeding or sleeping difficulties, which may add to the care-taking burden, and undermine parents' beliefs in their abilities to look after the child.

Speltz, Armsden and Clarren (1990) attempted to assess the relative contributions of these different variables to mothers' interactions with their infants. As in the study reported earlier, the infants were predominantly referred for craniofacial birth defects. Thirty-three mother–infant dyads were compared with a matched control group of healthy dyads. All mothers completed measures of stress (Loyd & Abidin 1985), general well-being and marital adjustment. They also rated their expectations for the child's future development and behaviour. In addition, mother-infant pairs were observed in both free play and more structured teaching interactions.

First of all, there were indications of greater stress and compromised self-competence among mothers of infants with craniofacial anomalies than among mothers of healthy infants. It was noted that the mothers felt their care-taking difficulties stemmed from their own inadequacies, rather than resulting from any difficulties in the infant. The authors point out that such attributions may serve an important function in promoting secure attachment between mother and infant by preserving positive feelings toward the child. By accepting responsibility themselves for any problems in caring for their children, these mothers were encouraged to persist in trying to improve the relationship with the infant. Perhaps they were successful. Despite these differences in reported stress and self-competence, there were no observable differences in interaction or affect in the play situations as a function of the health status of the child.

Speltz et al. (1990) concluded, however, that there is some evidence for a 'transactional' model of parental adjustment (Sameroff & Chandler 1975). Levels of stress and reported difficulties in parenting were unrelated to the severity of the child's condition, but mothers' reactions to the child appeared more dependent on variables such as her psychological status and marital functioning. Thus, mothers' responses to the child were determined by general environmental and social circumstances as much as by specifics of the condition. What is lacking in this study is any assessment from mothers themselves about their perceptions of the severity or extent of the disability. As will be argued in Chapter 5, ratings of this type are necessary to understand more fully the relationship between contextual and disease variables.

While the preschool period may be characterized by relative calm, families inevitably face some upheaval and disruption as the time for school approaches. Concern is likely since for many families, school attendance may be the first time that mother and child have been separated for any length of time, and parents are naturally concerned that teachers may not be aware of the child's health needs and potential vulnerability. For many it will also be the first time that explanations of the child's disease need to be given outside the immediate family, and this too may constitute some crisis. All mothers feel a mixture of pride and sorrow when their child first goes to school, and rattle around the house feeling empty. The transition from home to school can create specific practical anxieties for mothers of sick children, but one which has received little attention.

Long-term implications of chronic disease for later intellectual and social development

Does the onset of a chronic condition in infancy have a more negative effect on development than the onset of the same condition in later childhood? As was described in Chapter 1, Erikson (1959) suggested that the fundamental achievement in infancy is the development of a sense of *trust*. Given a warm caring environment, infants are expected to develop the essential ability to relate warmly to others, and this is assumed central to all later experiences. Conversely, a hostile or inconsistent experience during infancy is not conducive to the growth of a trusting relationship, and is associated with subsequent risks of suspicion and distrust. The experience of chronic disease would appear to jeopardize the growth of a basic trusting relationship. Infants are subjected to separations from parents and likely to experience care from a number of different nurses and other care-givers. A sense of trust is also likely to be violated as they experience painful treatments or diagnostic procedures.

During the toddler period, Erikson (1964) argued, the essential requirement was to gain a sense of *autonomy* rather than *shame*. Children need to understand that they have some control over their own behaviour. If parents do not allow their children to do what they can, or are overprotective, or require children to achieve before they are ready, a sense of shame or doubt is likely. Again, chronic disease is very likely to compromise attainments in this period, especially by increasing the probability that parents will overprotect or restrict their childrens' activities.

As a general criticism, Erikson's theory is hard to evaluate, and this applies as much to any assessment of the impact of chronic disease during infancy and the preschool period as during any other period. There are few, if any, standardized and acceptable measures of trust or autonomy suitable for this age-group. Given the difficulties of assessment in this age-group, it is perhaps not surprising that little research has any direct bearing on this question.

There are, however, indications that chronic conditions such as leukemia, diabetes, or epilepsy have particularly adverse effects on intellectual development when diagnosed in the infancy period. Treatments for many chronic diseases have at some time been associated with adverse side-effects, and these appear especially pronounced in younger children. Chemotherapy and radiation treatment have been linked to retarded cognitive development and academic difficulties in children with leukemia (Cousens *et al.* 1988; Eiser 1991). There is some evidence that these treatments, administered in the pre-school period, are potentially more damaging to normal cognitive development than the same treatments administered in middle- or late-childhood. For example, Eiser and Lansdown (1977) compared IQ scores of children treated for leukemia with those of a comparable group of healthy children. Differences between the groups were negligible for children treated after five years, but significant for those treated before five years, with those treated for leukemia having consistently lower scores.

One problem in interpreting these findings is that, although it is recognised that treatment is aggressive and potentially damaging, the children experience a number of other disadvantages. Not the least is a degree of social isolation, especially from other children, and this in itself may contribute to delays in social and academic functioning. Some children also experience physical limitations, through being hospitalised, or feeling too ill to run around and 'explore' in characteristic toddler fashion. There are, therefore, a number of possible explanations to account for the differences in functioning between children treated for leukemia and others over and above an explanation based on the side-effects of treatment.

However, similar findings have been reported for other conditions, particularly epilepsy (Dikmen, Mathews & Harley 1975) and diabetes (see Ryan 1990 for a review). Work investigating age of onset effects in relation to diabetes has been particularly consistent. Milberg, Hebben and Kaplan (1986) administered a comprehensive battery of neuropsychological tests to 125 children and adolescents with diabetes; their age at diagnosis ranged from 2 months to 14 years. Performance was compared against a control group of healthy children, most of whom were disease-free siblings. For the purposes of analyses, the children were divided into an 'early-onset' group (under five years on diagnosis) and a 'late-onset' group.

Those in the early onset group were found to be impaired in relation to healthy controls in every cognitive domain assessed.

> 'They learned new information less efficiently, they recalled less of that information after a 30-minute delay, they tended to distort or omit details when copying geometric designs, they made more errors on a number of different visual information-processing tasks and they performed more slowly (and less accurately) on tasks that required rapid responding. Not surprisingly, they also earned significantly lower scores on sub-tests from the Wechsler IQ scales, and performed more poorly on standardized measures of school achievement' (Ryan 1990, pp.67).

Further analyses suggested to the authors that in a number of cases, the magnitude of the differences between those in the early onset group and controls was clinically significant, and not attributable to chance fluctuations. On the criteria adopted, 24 per cent of the early onset group were clinically impaired, compared with 6 per cent of the late onset group and 6 per cent of the controls. Further, there were no significant differences between scores of the late onset group and their controls.

A related procedure was adopted by Rovet, Ehrlich and Hoppe (1987). However, the children in their study were younger, and a different test battery was employed. The sample consisted of 27 children in the early onset group (diagnosed before four years of age), 24 children with late onset diabetes, and 30 healthy sibling controls. Although there was an overall effect such that those with diabetes performed more poorly than those without, the children diagnosed before four years showed marked decrements in comparison with controls, especially on spatial tasks. At all ages, there was a difference in favour of the healthy controls on verbal tasks.

There are indications, then, that children who develop certain chronic conditions before five years of age, notably cancer, diabetes or epilepsy, are more likely to manifest cognitive impairments later in childhood compared with those diagnosed with the same conditions after five years. This age discrepancy suggests that school attendance is not the critical factor, since those diagnosed after beginning school would be expected to have poorer attendance records than children diagnosed and past the initial crisis before school entry.

A favoured hypothesis is that disease or treatment is more potentially damaging to the less mature brain (Moss, Nanis & Poplack 1981). Yet it is impossible to distinguish between this and the equally valid hypothesis that, by contracting a serious illness during early life, children miss out on valuable social and emotional experiences, which leaves them poorly prepared to face the world, so that learning is impaired. The picture is complicated because results point merely to statistical differences between groups of children; within any group, large variation can be observed, and most children function within defined normal limits. Some longitudinal studies which carefully trace changes in the social milieu in which the child develops, as well as chart fluctuations in cognitive functioning, are necessary.

Some early work concerned with the consequences of prematurity suggested that a degree of cognitive impairment was characteristic of all survivors. It was subsequently demonstrated that these effects were not inevitable, but modifiable through the social environment (Cohen & Parmelee 1983; Siegel et al. 1983). Specifically, children from more advantaged backgrounds showed no major, long-term adverse effects, whereas those from less privileged homes were more likely to have both cognitive and physical problems. Understanding the processes underlying the age of onset effects requires a much closer analysis of the relationship between disease, treatment and social environment.

Diagnosis of a chronic condition in early infancy is hard for parents, and requires them to develop considerable resourcefulness. Parents have very little time, sometimes none at all, to get to know their child just as a child, rather than as a child with cystic fibrosis, or haemophilia, or leukemia. The situation is very different when the child is believed to be healthy, but suddenly contracts a chronic condition in later childhood. In these situations, parents have come to expect that the child will develop normally, and they may have nurtured some hopes and expectations about the child's future and achievements. Diagnosis then, is a shock, but also violates expectations of normal growth, development and family life. In the following chapters, we will consider in more detail the impact of chronic disease during middle childhood and adolescence.

CHAPTER 3

The Importance of School for Normal Development

'I felt from the beginning that the only thing I had any control over was her schooling. I couldn't control the illness; I couldn't control the drugs, but I could make sure she enjoyed school and did well there. It's not enough for me that she's alive; I want to feel she has a good life too. That's why it's so hard for me now; she is off treatment, but she's not the same child. She used to be very independent, was always happy to go with other people or stay the night with friends. Now she just clings on. And school is a disaster. She has put on weight, and has some lung damage; so she's no good at games. I was a teacher; I know it's really important to be good at games. If friends from school come round, she wanders off after 10 minutes and plays by herself, and her younger brothers are better at everything' (Mother of 9-year-old child treated for leukemia).

The importance of school for children with chronic disease cannot be underestimated. As described by the mother above, it is often the yardstick by which the impact of the disease is assessed. It is generally considered advantageous for children to return to school as soon as possible after diagnosis. In the short term, it enables them to resume old friendships and re-establish themselves amongst peers. The school environment offers children opportunities for play and social interaction, as well as enabling them to participate in sports activities and outings. A speedy return to school also minimizes the amount of lesson time lost reducing, it is hoped, the extent to which children fall behind others in academic work. Return to school is also important for other family members. Apart from signalling that the child can lead a relatively normal life, it enables parents to pick up their own lives again. For many parents, it is important that they are able to return to work as quickly as possible. Caring for a sick child is expensive. Many firms do not offer substantial benefits or paid leave of absence, and it is almost impossible for those who are self-employed to take time off work. In the longer term, return to school is necessary so that the child has as good opportunities for future employment as possible.

Weitzman (1984) summarised the advantages of schooling more formally. He argued that school attendance is necessary so that the child becomes aware of social and cultural norms and develops a sense of belonging and identity with these norms and values. School allows the child to develop a sense of belonging to a wider social group than the immediate family. Opportunities arise which enable the child to develop social and interactive skills, both with adults and peers. According to Erikson (1964), the attainment of a sense of accomplishment is important during this period. It is in the school environment that most opportunities for accomplishment arise, as does exposure to stressful situations. Recognising and coping with stress is an integral part of a successful school career, and often assumed to play a major role in determining adjustment in adult life.

Fowler, Johnson and Atkinson (1985) also stressed the importance of school attendance in promoting child independence and autonomy. They suggest that one of the most important tasks of childhood is the move beyond the family to the school community where academic achievement, social competence and regular attendance are major goals.

In practice, some children find the return to school after diagnosis to be more difficult than expected. Extended absences around the time of diagnosis may mean that the child starts at some disadvantage, both academically and socially. The class would have begun new topics in many subjects, and the sick child can experience constant difficulty in making up the lost work. Healthy children may feel confused about the illness and its implications, and this confusion may be reflected in teasing and rejection. It also needs to be remembered that the sick child does not return to class as exactly the same person as before the illness. There may be some changes in physical appearance which may be particularly disturbing to small children. Emotionally and mentally there may be some changes too. The experience of hospital, treatment and extensive interactions with adults may change the sick child. This may be reflected in heightened emotionality and tendencies to behave in younger ways. Some chronically sick children may react by becoming adept at 'mothering' others, and enjoy looking after smaller children. In contrast, they are sometimes uncomfortable and ill at ease with their own peer group.

While some children respond badly to chronic illness, perhaps behaving in very baby-like ways or expecting others to make allowances for them, others seem to gain considerable maturity. In knowing that they have coped and come through the initial stages of the illness, the children may have gained some insight and autonomy in comparison with their healthier class-mates. Chronic disease can act as a stimulus to the promotion of psychological growth and mature, autonomous functioning.

Childrens' experiences on return to school after diagnosis or long absences

Almost all teachers have a child with a chronic condition in their class at some point during their careers. Few feel comfortable with the situation. Younger teachers especially are unlikely to have any personal contact with sick children, and even less likely to have experienced any formal training about their needs. Children with chronic disease require varying degrees of practical help during the school day. For example, at the simplest level, children with asthma may need to have access to their inhaler occasionally. Schools vary in their attitudes to this, with some happy to ensure that the inhaler is kept near to hand and accessible at all times. Other schools require that all medications are locked in a Head-teacher's office, with the result that inhalers may not be immediately available in an emergency. At the other extreme, children with motor difficulties may require considerable practical help, often solved by having specific individuals or groups of children responsible for helping the child move around the school. Considerable organisation is also required for pupils with cystic fibrosis. Many of these children require physiotherapy three times a day. They must therefore routinely go home for lunch, or arrangements be made for a school-nurse or teacher's aide to administer the treatment.

A child's view of asthma

'It's O.K. having asthma. You feel dizzy and wheezy. The worse thing is the attacks. You get very worked up about having the attacks. Once I got so worked up I tripped over the table and went to the wrong drawer and everybody stared at me. It's very frustrating. Lots of people die of attacks, but it stops when you're 18. You can pass asthma on then, and you don't have it' (Charlie, aged 8 years).

'Asthma is a disorder of the tracheobronchial tree in which there is recurrent, at least partially reversible generalized obstruction to the airflow. It is commonly manifested by cough and expiratory distress and classically by expiratory wheezing. Overt wheezing does not have to occur, however, and the major manifestations may be cough' (Pearlman 1984, p.459).

Asthma is often considered to be the least serious of the chronic conditions of childhood, and in some cases it can cause few and infrequent problems. A wide range of stimuli can precipitate asthma attacks in vulnerable individuals (Reed & Townley 1983). Environmental and air pollutants are coming under increasing scrutiny. Incomplete combustion of fossil fuels and resultant smog, and the effects of ultraviolet irradiation on car exhaust fumes are the biggest problem. Cigarette smoke has also been implicated.

Other precipitants include exercise, infections and emotions. Many children experience exercise-induced asthma, particularly when participating in sports involving vigorous exercise in cold, dry conditions. Some care needs to be taken in choice of exercise for children with asthma. Playing rugby or ice-skating may be less advisable than a swim in a warm pool. Children are also more likely to experience attacks when they are run down, or have colds and 'flu, suggesting that some care should be taken to isolate children from contagious conditions. Crying and laughing can also precipitate attacks in some children. Allergies to pollens, house dust, animals or feathers and some foods are also common, and frequently have an inherited component.

Diagnosis is often based on the child's or parents' reports about the incidence and nature of respiratory attacks rather than observation of symptoms and experiences. Confirmatory diagnosis entails two steps; provocation challenge and response assessment. The first involves presenting the patient with samples of some of the stimulants described above. The patient's skin may be pricked with a needle containing a small amount of the stimulant. A more direct 'bronchial challenge' involves the inhalation of minute quantities of stimulant and examination of the consequent activity of the airways. The second involves measurement of respiratory function under defined conditions.

Asthma is characterised by its intermittent nature, its variability and reversibility. Most children experience attacks on an intermittent basis; an episode of frequent attacks can be followed by a period of months or years when no attacks occur. Asthma also varies in terms of severity. In the mildest attacks, children may simply experience a slight tightening of the chest or slight wheeze. At the other extreme, an attack can be so severe as to result in death. Asthma is reversible, in that between attacks children's breathing can be quite normal. Treatments can be palliative in that children require treatment only during specific periods when attacks are pronounced. Other children require continuous treatment to control the condition.

How do children who have asthma feel about their condition? The experience of breathlessness can be very frightening, both for the child and the for parent who must watch. Children can resent the restrictions imposed by their susceptibility to specific precipitants; they can feel very put out because they cannot go to the zoo with the rest of the class, and very unhappy where attacks appear to be precipitated by the family pet. Many particularly dislike being made to feel different from their school friends, and fear attacks in school and looking a fool.

Lack of information is translated directly to anxiety and doubts about how best to treat the child. Much unnecessary concern occurs because teachers fear the child will be ill in school, and they lack confidence to deal with the unexpected. Teachers are naturally worried about how to deal with emergencies, such as an asthma attack or an epileptic fit. As a result, they may well overestimate the probable incidence of such events. They face dilemmas as to whether to encourage the child to take part in all activities or let them take a back-seat. They may feel confused about the long-term aims of teaching for children with potentially limited life-expectancies. Teachers may therefore modify their expectations for sick children, redefining the purpose of school so that academic achievements are seen to be less important than for healthy children (Eiser & Town 1987).

There is considerable empirical evidence that children can find the return to school difficult. For example, Chesler, Paris and Barbarin (1986) surveyed parents of children with cancer, and found that 51 per cent reported that their child had experienced some difficulties. These largely could be accounted for by school absences, creating difficulties with school work and slowing academic progress. Other problems were caused by teasing or rejection by peers. While 55 per cent of parents felt that school staff had been helpful in re-integrating their child into the classroom, the remainder had experienced unhelpful behaviour from school staff. Teachers' behaviours which were judged to be specially helpful included caring, treating the child as normal, giving special academic help and keeping parents well informed about what was happening in the classroom. Unhelpful behaviours included insensitivity, over-protectiveness and refusing to acknowledge the reality of the situation, (telling parents that everything was fine). Differences between teachers in terms of the extent to which they were judged to be helpful were unrelated to the age of the children.

Most research attention has focussed on return to school of children with cancer. Certainly, there are good reasons to think that the experience might be difficult for them. They must return after what may have been a relatively long absence, during which time they would have been diagnosed, and experienced hospital admission, chemotherapy and radiotherapy. These treatments themselves are likely to make children feel physically very ill. In addition, they may well have been made aware of the potentially life-threatening nature of their illness, and the long-term aspects of treatment. As a result, children may be forced to return to school looking very different from before, perhaps having gained considerable weight and almost certainly having lost much of their hair. Difficulties are likely to be aggravated through the continuing need to attend out-patient clinics, further jeopardizing a completely normal return to school.

Extended absence (Deasey-Spinetta & Spinetta 1980; Eiser 1980), teasing (Greene 1975) and sometimes extreme cases of school phobia (Lansky et al. 1975) have all been reported. In the study by Lansky et al. (1975), it was noted that some 10 per cent of those returning to school immediately following treatment for cancer showed evidence of school phobia, including school refusal and extreme clinging and dependence. Eiser (1980) found that school absence was very high in the six months following diagnosis, but improved steadily over longer periods of time. According to teachers' estimates, only 33 per cent of children with cancer had attendance rates which were comparable with the rest of the class. Deasey-Spinetta and Spinetta (1980) asked teachers to judge a child in their class with cancer in relation to one other healthy peer. Those with cancer were rated no differently in terms of their willingness to attend school, the extent to which they were teased by others or degree of dependent behaviour. However, they were described as being lower in energy levels and were reported to have more difficulty in concentrating and completing projects than other children in the class. They were also rated as emotionally inhibited and less likely to express their feelings.

Given the improvements in treatment protocols developed in recent years to manage childhood cancer, it might be hoped that childrens' experiences have changed for the better. There is only tangential infor-mation to support this view. Larcombe et al. (1990) compared the school experiences of 51 children with cancer with that of 66 with other chronic diseases, including renal disease, cardiac and orthopedic conditions. Children from both groups experienced some difficulties on returning to school, but these were greatest for those with cancer and least for those with orthopedic conditions. Physical problems, especially nausea, tired-ness and lack of mobility were reported to create more difficulties than being behind in school work. Some children, especially in the group with cancer, missed a large amount of schooling, but these were generally necessitated by genuine hospital appointments or periods of infection.

Much attention has focussed on childhood cancer because it is a highly visible condition, as well as being emotive and potentially life-threatening. Children with renal disease may also become bloated-look-

QUEEN MARGARET COLLEGE LIBRARY

ing, or develop excess body hair as a result of drug treatment. Yet they have received virtually no attention in the research literature. The difficulties faced by children with other chronic conditions may be extensive, although necessarily of a different kind. Those children with cystic fibrosis who have to spend lunch-time having physiotherapy rather than playing with the others, are clearly likely to feel singled out and different. Children with asthma or diabetes, for example, may be responsible themselves for administering some aspects of the treatment, both outside and within the school setting. For children with diabetes, juggling snacks before exercise may involve them in embarrassing explanations which continually set them apart from class-mates in a way that is not experienced by those with cancer. Children with asthma, also, may need to take prophylactic treatment before exercise, or at other times of the day. Again, demands associated with self-care in these conditions may have the effect of aggravating differences between children with chronic disease and others.

Absences

Despite these potential difficulties, it is rare that children with other chronic diseases show as extreme cases of school phobia as has been documented for those with cancer (Lansky et al. 1975). Yet there is plenty of evidence of increased school absence; in diabetes (Bradbury & Smith 1983), in epilepsy (Holdsworth & Whitmore 1974), in haemophilia (Lineberger 1981; Markova, MacDonald & Forbes 1980; Woolf et al. 1989) and asthma (Hill, Standen & Tattersfield 1989). From the results of larger scale, comparative studies, it is possible to see that children with some conditions experience more frequent absences and consequently more interrupted schooling than others. Fowler, Johnson and Atkinson (1985) contacted the families of 270 children suffering from one of 11 different conditions. The mean number of days absence for the total group was 16 days compared with less than seven days for healthy children over the same period. Those with cystic fibrosis, sickle-cell disease, arthritis, haemophilia or spina bifida averaged the most absences.

As might be expected, children with chronic diseases are potentially at some disadvantage in school, and this is most obviously reflected in a tendency toward poorer school attendance compared with healthy children. There are many possible explanations for these poor atten-dance records. The children are likely to experience bouts of genuine illness associated with their condition, or perhaps be more susceptible to minor infections. Of necessity, they miss some school in order to attend out-patient clinics or other hospital appointments. Teachers are sometimes skeptical about how genuine absences are. Boys with hae-mophilia for example, miss school to attend hospital, because of bleeding episodes and for general illness symptoms (Markova, MacDonald & Forbes 1980). Parents may feel inclined to keep children at home in case of infection. Eiser (1980), for example, in a survey of 41 children with leukemia, found that three had been removed from the normal school setting by their parents, who had successfully organised home tuition for the child. In all cases, parents had taken the decision about removal from school in order to reduce the risk of infection. Similar decisions are often taken by parents of children with cystic fibrosis, again justified on the grounds of the child's heightened vulnerability to infections. At least as far as children with asthma are concerned, we have found that parents perceive their children to be highly vulnerable to everyday infection, frequently describing their children as 'picking up everything that's going' or 'always first to catch whatever's around', (Eiser, Eiser, Town & Tripp 1991a). Beliefs like these may contribute substantially to parents' decisions to keep their child away from school more often than teachers or doctors would consider necessary.

School absence is certainly not simply related to the seriousness of the disease. Social factors and parents' attitudes to school generally play a part. Thus, Anderson *et al.* (1983) found that the extent to which children with asthma attended school regularly was determined less by the severity of their condition than the extent to which the family had adequate resources. School attendance was related to the number of children in the family, (better attendance with fewer children); mother's access to a car, and whether or not she worked outside the home. Charlton *et al.* (1991) compared school absence rates in children treated for cancer, chronic (renal disease, cardiac conditions, asthma and other nondefined conditions) or orthopedic conditions. Absence rates were most clearly predicted from the condition, with children with cancer having highest absence rates. During the initial phases of treatment, median absence rates for children with cancer was 91 days, for those with chronic conditions median absence rates were 29.5 days, and the comparable figure for those with orthopedic conditions was 15 days. The authors reported increased absences for non-illness reasons to be higher in girls than boys. The only factor apart from illness which was associated with children's absence rates was mothers' level of education; attendance was better among those whose mother was educated beyond 18 years. These women may value education more highly themselves, and therefore foster attitudes in their families about the importance of education, or it may be that they are more able to understand information about the disease. Increased understanding may enable them to balance more effectively the potentially positive effects that may occur for the child in regularly attending school against the risks of infection.

Weitzman (1986) also notes that many absences are not justified, and suggests that these can often be attributed to inaccurate beliefs about the illness and its consequences. In a survey of mothers of children with asthma, Eiser *et al.* (1991b) found that some women reported keeping their children at home on days when they thought an attack *might* occur, whether or not the child showed signs of illness before school.

Whatever the reasons for school absence, the real question must be with the consequences of the absences. It might be expected that school absence would be associated with lowered educational attainments, reduced examination successes and ultimately less successful integration in the work-force. We might also expect social consequences, with children feeling isolated and poorly integrated with the rest of the school. Teachers, and other children, may feel tempted to treat chronically sick children differently and expect altered levels of achievement or behaviour. In the next section, we will examine the evidence for these assumptions.

Teachers' expectations and behaviour

Teachers face many dilemmas in dealing with children who have a chronic or fatal condition in the class-room. Many have little personal experience of such illnesses, or the experience that they do have may well be negative. Although many people have known someone with cancer, this experience may not fit them well for handling a child with the disease. This is due to the differences in the etiology and prognosis of many adult cancers compared with those affecting children as well as the wide variability in outcome of different cancers affecting children. In cases of hereditary conditions, such as haemophilia, previous experience may lead adults to expect greater difficulties and more interrupted school and social lives than should be expected for the majority of patients to-day. Thus, personal experience may be of limited value in helping teachers to know how to respond to sick children in the class-room and may even on occasions be associated with unnecessarily negative and inappropriate expectations.

If personal experience is of limited help, it is particularly unfortunate that professional training is rarely adequate either. Few professional training courses offer adequate guidance. Teachers are therefore dependent on subsequent in-service and professional development training. Courses concerned with teaching chronically sick children need to compete with a vast number of other issues, many of which are likely to be seen as more widely relevant.

Yet it is clear that teachers could well benefit from some discussion of the issues raised in teaching sick children. Not least is an assessment of the meaning of school to the sick child, and what can realistically be achieved, in both the short- and long-term. Teachers need to consider ways of handling parents and sometimes helping them set realistic goals for their children. In addition, they must establish ways of educating themselves regarding the implications of the condition. A real practical concern is how to ensure that they are up-dated as necessary about changes in childrens' health. Even parents who are reliable informants on diagnosis may forget to update teachers about changes in the child's condition, or fail to realise that the information they give to one teacher is not always relayed to other staff, particularly when children change classes. Not least, teachers need to work out details of information about the disease that need to be given to other children in the class, and how to respond to questions about the disease, especially where deteriorating or fatal conditions are involved. A teacher who was working in the same school that her child attended was confronted with the task of dealing with the school's distress when her own child died from cancer.

'When Gary died, the whole school mourned; teachers, dinner-ladies, the caretaker, the children. But nobody talked to the children; we were all too busy dealing with our own emotions.'

Unfortunately, it is clear that many teachers lack understanding about the changes and improvements in treatment of many childhood diseases, often believing that prognosis is poorer than suggested by current statistics. In some cases, this can be attributed to a lack of willingness on the part of parents (and sometimes the child) to involve the school very effectively in relevant information about the condition. For example, Bradbury and Smith (1983) found that teachers were uninformed about diabetes, even where they were teaching a child with the disease. They generally expressed many concerns about appropriate behaviour, and the extent to which the child should be encouraged to participate fully in the curriculum. In cases where the child's parents also have diabetes, difficulties can be aggravated further. Kirk and Savage (1985) found that these families needed special support. Parents' knowledge was often poor, and they tended to adopt over-anxious or highly protective behaviours towards their children. Adults with diabetes may become very lax in their own self-care behaviours, and are therefore poor role models for their children. Worries about complications and feelings of guilt about 'passing on' the condition aggravated parents' concerns.

There can also be a reluctance on the part of medical personnel to provide much in the way of appropriate information for schools. Walker (1984) argues that this 'lack of realistic information (from the Pediatrician) can actually hurt the child's progress through school; since it may result in an inappropriate educational placement, the denial of a necessary related service, or over-protective attitudes and behaviours on the part of uninformed school personnel' (p.222).

The combined effects of reluctance on the part of parent and medical personnel to involve teachers consistently in details of the disease or its management results in an understandable lack of information and uncertainty about how to treat the child (Eiser & Town 1987), as well as fostering some inappropriate and sometimes derogatory stereotypes. Stern & Arenson (1989) asked medical students and undergraduates to rate hypothetical children described as healthy or in remission from leukemia on a number of bipolar scales. Children in remission were rated as less sociable, less cognitively competent, less behaviourally active, less well-behaved, smaller and less likely to adjust well to the future than healthy children. These ratings were made by medical students (with some familiarity with the consequences of leukemia for adjustment) and undergraduates (with little or no formal experience). The authors concluded that such negative stereotypes pervade the thinking of many adults in society, and are likely to jeopodize the potential adjustment of children treated for leukemia.

Eiser and Town (1987) surveyed 147 experienced teachers about their knowledge of four conditions (asthma, diabetes, cancer and epilepsy). Knowledge of all four conditions was minimal, and many misconceptions were identified. For example, over half the teachers believed that emotional problems between mother and child pre-dated asthma. Teachers were most concerned about their own inabilities to handle medical emergencies and the impact on other children of witnessing episodes of ill-health such as asthma attacks or epileptic seizures. For the most part, teachers were unsure about what to expect of sick children, and requested some guide-lines as to what children could safely and reasonably be expected to do.

Bevis and Taylor (1990) also reported that many teachers knew very little about one of the most common chronic conditions, asthma; and for the most part they were aware of their relative ignorance. Only 27 per cent knew that playing games in a cold wind could provoke an asthma attack and only 34 per cent would recognize that wheezing after games was a worrying sign. Although there was variability in teachers' awareness of asthma, the overall school policy regarding the storage and use of medicants in school was often confused and unhelpful. Barely half the teachers involved in the study allowed children to keep their inhaler with them at all times. Concerns about over-dosing, loss, use by other children, addiction, paranoia and 'conflict with school policy' were cited as reasons in support of these policies.

The need to inform schools and educate teachers about a child's medical history has to be weighed against the risk of 'labelling' and compromising a potentially normal school environment (Levenson and Cooper 1984). Together with arguments about confidentiality, this has often been taken as justification on the part of parents and medical professionals to withhold information from schools. Yet parents themselves endorse the notion that schools should be informed. In a rare survey of parents' opinions, Andrews (1991) notes that parents of children with a range of chronic conditions felt it was appropriate that schools should be informed, particularly about physical aspects of the disease and treatment. They least strongly believed that schools needed information about the emotional consequences of the condition. While parents recognised their own responsibility to inform schools, they felt that physicians were the most appropriate informants about physical aspects, possible emergencies, and side-effects of medication. Although the sample was drawn from a university clinic and was skewed in favour of a more educated sample, the results suggest that these parents would welcome closer liaisons between schools, hospital and home. Satisfactory coordination between home, hospital and school may prove more difficult to achieve where conflicts exist prior to the diagnosis.

Many specialist centres now appoint liaison nurses whose role it is to inform schools about the disease and advise over the impact on school life. It is increasingly common that such liaison nurses are attached to specialist centres, particularly those caring for children with cancer, diabetes or cystic fibrosis. These nurses clearly have an important role in ensuring that the child's school life is as normal as possible. Yet this is financially viable only in relation to large centres. Many children are treated from smaller or less well funded centres, where the lack of liaison nurses means that opportunities for misunderstanding and communication between school, hospital and home, are rife.

Educational adjustment

For some children with chronic disease, there are good reasons to suppose that educational achievements may be somewhat compromised. For example, drugs used in the treatment of epilepsy are thought to be associated with organic damage. Schlieper *et al.* (1991) reported that theophylline, routinely used in the treatment of asthma, was associated with no side-effects for the majority of children, but was linked with academic and behavioural disturbances in a minority. Children with cancer are treated with toxic drugs (for example methotrexate) and cranial irradiation, both of which have been linked with residual organic damage (Eiser 1991). In some cases, the disease itself may be associated with damage and this appears to apply especially to very young children. Thus, as discussed in Chapter 2, children with diabetes who experience repeated episodes of ketoacidosis are reported to show reduced levels of functioning in comparison with children with diabetes who do not experience a similar number of episodes (Ack, Miller & Weil 1961; Rovet, Ehrlich & Hoppe 1987).

For the most part, systematic study of educational achievements or intellectual development more generally has been most prolific in relation to children with leukemia or diabetes. This interest in leukemia reflects the fact that some aspects of routine treatments are associated with serious side-effects and complications. In the 1960s and '70s, it was found that chemotherapy alone was of limited value in long-term control of the disease. This was attributed to a protective mechanism in the brain, which decreased the amount of drug allowed into brain tissue. The result was that many patients experienced Central Nervous System (CNS) disease, and consequently, very poor prognosis. Treatment directly of the CNS is generally considered essential to increase the chances of long-term survival. The significant improvements in prognosis over the last 30 or so years are attributed to the introduction of CNS radiotherapy as part of routine induction treatment (Poplack 1988).

This treatment is controversial, however, since it involves irradiation of healthy central nervous system (CNS) tissue. The aim of treatment is essentially prophylactic; that is, it is intended to reduce the *probability* of CNS disease in the future, rather than cure an established problem. Added to this is the fact that many parents expressed concern about side-effects of the treatment, and a minority of children seemed to develop varying degrees of cognitive malfunction. To establish a single cause of such malfunction is impossible. Children with leukemia face many difficulties; to some extent it is a remarkable achievement that the majority survive with so few psychological handicaps. They miss considerable amounts of schooling; they often feel unwell as a result of chemotherapy; teachers and parents may limit their activities; at times they look different from other children. Small wonder if school progress does not always match that of healthy peers and siblings.

A proportion of published research has not identified any intellectual deficits in children treated for leukemia (see Eiser 1991; Madan-Swain & Brown 1991 for reviews). The magnitude of the deficits reported in other studies varies considerably. The results of a meta-analysis published by Cousens *et al.* (1988) suggested that greater decrements occur (1) among children treated by CNS irradiation before five years of age compared with children receiving the same treatment after this age; (2) when comparisons are made with healthy controls rather than children with other cancers; and (3) increase the longer the time since diagnosis.

Inconsistencies in this literature can be attributed to difficulties in controlling a number of variables, including the current health status of the child. Standard protocols involve two years' chemotherapy, after which time it is hoped that the child is 'cured'. During treatment, when the child is receiving chemotherapy and experiencing other procedures as well, it is perhaps to be expected that some deficits in functioning might be identified compared with well children. Yet, given the rapidly improving survival rates, it is important that children recover after cessation of therapy, and achieve normal levels of functioning. The literature reviewed so far sometimes fails to distinguish between children currently receiving treatment and those who have completed treatment. Increasingly, attention is turning to long-term survivors, for two reasons. Clinically, it is important to establish whether individuals who have survived cancer treatment as children show any long term deficits in functioning which might jeopardize their social or occupational opportunities. Theoretically, by studying this group, it should be possible to understand the processes whereby radiation and chemotherapy affect cognitive functioning, and the mechanisms whereby recovery occurs in the event of organic impairment.

Peckham et al. (1988) studied 23 children who had been treated at least eight years earlier for leukemia. They were still somewhat behind in reading and mathematics, and also experienced difficulties in attention, concentration, memory and comprehension. Yet the extent to which the children evidenced such difficulties varied enormously, and was markedly reduced where families and schools had been able to offer remedial help and support. Other work, (Feldman 1980) also suggests that children from families of higher educational background were more likely than those from other backgrounds to improve academic performance on return to school.

Related conclusions were drawn by Mulhern et al. (1989). Children who had been treated by cranial irradiation and lived in one-parent families were most vulnerable to school-related problems and somatic complaints of unknown origin. Together these studies suggest that long-term survivors of childhood cancer are at some risk of intellectual and social development, but the degree of risk can be off-set by sensitive schooling and adequate family support. Other work suggests there is an increased risk of physical side-effects, including growth problems, lung damage and susceptibility to secondary cancers. For all these reasons, there is considerable concern that long-term survivors should be offered comprehensive follow-up and surveillance. This needs to be balanced, however, against the wishes of individuals, who may resent being constantly reminded that they once had a life-threatening condition.

Although it is recognised that many children with cancer experience disruptions in their schooling and may be offered some remedial help, it is not clear that this is always successful or indeed appropriate for their specific needs. Educational interventions tend to mirror general approaches offered to children presenting with a variety of learning dis-

abilities, and are not necessarily tailored to children who are of potentially normal or above average ability, but disadvantaged by chronic
disease and repeated hospitalizations and school absence. The rift between research and practice is wide in this context. The implications
from research findings are that children may benefit from specific remedial education programmes designed to enhance memory functioning
or problem solving. Instead, they are most usually offered 'extra' help
along with other slow-learners; most frequently a teacher's aide is
assigned to the whole class for a small proportion of the week. There
have been no systematic efforts to assess if this type of intervention has
any beneficial effect at all. Lack of theoretical understanding of the
processes whereby radiotherapy distorts normal cognitive growth also
limit the development of appropriate remedial interventions.

Social adjustment

In reading the literature, it is almost possible to feel that attention to
children's school attendance and achievements is disproportional to that
concerned with the social or emotional sequelae of disease. This can be
attributable to some extent to the fact that attendance and attainments
are more easily measurable than social functioning, and this appeals to
those wanting more 'objective' indices of adjustment. Attendance can
be quantified in absolute terms, as can reading skill or I.Q. There is much
less agreement about how to measure social and emotional variables.
Perhaps also this bias reflects the concerns of medical staff and parents.
It is possible to discuss a child's poor school progress, and come to some
decision about practical steps that can be taken. In contrast, it is more
difficult to pass judgment about children's social behaviour, and harder
still to see what can be done to change the situation. Judgments of these
issues are dependent on one's frame of reference, and are far less
tangible, or amenable to intervention.

Although there has been a large amount of research concerned with
'adjustment' in chronically sick children, few have really tackled the
issue of what it means to be adjusted to a chronic or life-threatening
condition. Distinctions have been made between adjustment to regular
everyday demands which are shared by sick and healthy children, and
adjustment to demands which are specific to the disease and its treatment. In the former category, adjustment may refer to the child's school
attendance and participation in age appropriate social and leisure activities. In the latter category would be included the child's adjustment
or acceptance of hospitalization, preparedness to keep out-patient appointments, and cooperation with self-care and home management of
the disease. Pless and Pinkerton (1975) also make the point that adjustment is a dynamic concept; it is affected by changes in the child's health

as well as subject to fluctuations in relation to school or family experiences. Thus, adjustment should not be seen to be a linear dimension such that children can be neatly allocated to different end-points; rather adjustment is a constantly changing and elusive phenomenum. Neither is it altogether clear that adjustment manifests itself in the same way for all children, regardless of age, gender or specifics of the condition.

Adjustment is generally defined operationally, and is thus inferred from assessments of behavioural psychopathology, self-concept, aggression and loneliness, among many other characteristics. However, one of the most frequently cited instruments is the Child Behaviour Checklist (CBCL) (Achenbach & Edelbrock 1983). According to Perrin, Stein and Drotar (1991), 12 of 20 studies concerned with adjustment in chronically sick children and published during the period 1987–1989 used the CBCL. The original measure was designed to obtain reports from parents about their child's behaviour. The measure was subsequently developed to be suitable for teacher assessment (TRF), and a further measure is suitable for completion by the children themselves (Youth Self-Report (YSR)) (Achenbach & Edelbrock 1986). The instrument is, however, coming under increasing criticism, especially with regard to its suitability as an assessment tool for children with chronic disease (Sandberg, Meyer-Bahlberg & Yager 1991; Walker et al. 1990; Perrin, Stein & Drotar 1991).

Perrin, Stein and Drotar (1991) identified three limitations in using the Child Behaviour Checklist with groups of chronically sick children. These include (1) possible bias in interpreting questions about physical symptoms, (2) limited sensitivity to mild adjustment problems and (3) incomplete and potentially misleading assessment of social competence.

With respect to the first reservation, it should be noted that the CBCL includes a number of items to assess physical symptoms. Two items refer to specific diagnoses (asthma and allergies). Eight other items refer to the occurrence of physical symptoms without known medical cause (e.g. eye problems, vomiting, stomach-aches). As Perrin, Stein and Drotar (1991) point out, it is rarely possible to be certain whether or not symptoms such as these really have no known cause or are more directly attributable to an organic condition. Since children with chronic disease may have physical symptoms as a result of their disease or because of treatment, they are in any case likely to have elevated scores. This is likely to be reflected in increased scores on subscales measuring 'somatic complaints' and 'internalizing problems', as well as on the total score. (A higher incidence of internalizing problems was indeed found among children with arthritis in the study reported by Wallander et al. 1988).

'A similar problem is raised by items that refer to physical symptoms that may suggest psychogenic disturbance but which are also symptoms of particular chronic physical disorders. For example "nervous movements or twitching" or "stares blankly" may reflect a seizure disorder, "constipated" or "wets self" may accompany spina bifida, and "feels dizzy" may be a symptom of hypoglycemia in children with diabetes. Other more ambiguous items of this sort include "lacks energy" and "speech problem". Inclusion of such items could again lead to findings suggesting spuriously high rates of behavioural disturbance in children with a chronic illness' (Perrin, Stein & Drotar 1991, p.414).

A second problem refers to the suitability of the CBCL for the assessment of mild behaviour problems of the kind to be expected in children with chronic disease. Instead, the instrument was designed to assess psychopathology. Given that recent theoretical approaches emphasise coping and adjustment in chronically sick children, it is important that assessment instruments should reflect this theoretical stance. The continued focus on psychopathology and deficits is not justified from either a theoretical or methodological perspective.

Third, the items used to assess social competence tend to measure accomplishment, and participation in activities rather than competence in social interaction. 'Several items assess outcomes such as the level of activity in sports and clubs that may be limited by illness, physical handicap, special transportation requirements, doctors' appointments, and medication needs. The fact that some children with a chronic illness are unable to participate in certain social activities solely because of their condition does not mean that they are less socially competent' (Perrin, Stein & Drotar 1991, p.416).

It is unfortunate that so much work in this area has relied on inappropriate measures of adjustment in chronically sick children, with an emphasis so much toward maladjustment rather than coping or adjustment. Partly as a result of limited availability of good assessment instruments, there is much variability in the reported incidence and degree of maladjustment in chronically sick children. Wallander *et al.* (1988) attributes this to a lack of methodological rigor, and notes especially the different conclusions to be drawn depending on whether a population or cross-sectional approach is adopted. Population- based approaches tend to include representative samples of children suffering from a wide-range of chronic conditions. These studies point consistently to maladjustment in chronically sick children, both in relation to healthy peers (Eiser 1990) and siblings (Cadman *et al.* 1988).

Advocates of this approach argue that it is possible to identify subgroups of chronically sick children at disproportionate risk. In the study reported by Cadman, Boyle, Offord and Szatmari (1987), it was possible to survey 3294 randomly selected children. The data were presented in such a way that it is possible to quantify maladjustment risks for the total group, and separately for subgroups of the population of chronically sick children. For children with chronic disease alone, the age and gender adjusted odds ratio for one or more psychiatric disorders was 2.1. For those with chronic disease and physical disability, this ratio increased to 3.4. The survey points to increases in risk of neurotic disorders for all children, and of social isolation and loneliness for those with physical disability. Population studies point also to the increased vulnerability for children with diseases involving neurological (Rutter, Tizard & Whitmore 1970; Breslau & Marshall 1985), and sensory impairments (Pless 1984).

In contrast to the population-based studies, there is much greater variability in the conclusions to be drawn from cross-sectional studies. There are many reasons for this, including differences in disease groups studied and methods of assessment employed. In addition, sample sizes tend to be small, and are often drawn from a single clinic or hospital setting. Thus, results may reflect specific policies rather than be applicable to a general population. In that much research is conducted from prestigious medical centres or teaching hospitals, it may be that much of this work tends to underestimate the degree and prevalence of maladjustment in general populations.

Regardless of the particular methods employed, at least two theoretical perspectives can be identified, (see Chapter 1 for an initial discussion). According to the 'non-categorical' approach (Stein & Jessop 1982, Wallander et al. 1988), there are many more similarities than differences between children with various conditions, with the result that identifiable differences in qualitative aspects of maladjustment are unlikely. Thus, general increases in practical stress or care-taking demands, the need to interact with medical staff and uncertainties about prognosis are general disadvantages shared by all children with chronic disease and their families. This approach is in contrast particularly with earlier assumptions that specific characteristics were associated with the onset and experience of different diseases. (Thus, Dunbar (1954) argued that patients with diabetes could be distinguished from those with other illnesses in that they were characterized by dependence–independence conflicts, poor sexual adjustment, anxiety, depression and paranoia. Others have argued that childhood asthma is related to conflict in the mother-child relationship; (a belief that we found to be still widespread among many teachers, Eiser & Town 1987)). The search for specific personality types characterizing particular conditions is no longer generally in vogue, but neither is there substantial empirical evidence for the validity of a completely non-categorical approach. In part, this is a consequence of the necessary research not being conducted. Although population-based studies do include children with a variety of conditions, they do not generally include measures of sufficient sensitivity to detect subtle differences between groups. They also tend to be based on measures of deficit or maladjustment, rather than coping and adjustment. On the other hand, cross-sectional studies may well include a wider range of measures with the aim of identifying coping resources as well as difficulties, but they rarely include comparisons of children with different conditions.

A limited body of research points to the general disadvantage that is associated with chronic disease, and additional problems that can occur in children with specific conditions. For example, Wallander *et al.* (1988) asked mothers to rate the adjustment of their children using the Child behaviour Checklist. The children suffered from one of six conditions (diabetes, spina bifida, haemophilia, obesity, arthritis and cerebral palsy). Mothers rated the total group of sick children as less well adjusted than a control group of mothers rated their healthy children. Those with diabetes, spina bifida, haemophilia and obesity were not distinguishable from each other. However, those with arthritis showed fewer 'externalizing' problems (e.g. less likely to threaten people, swear, or demand attention) and those with cerebral palsy scored lower on the social competence sub-scale.

Using a comparable methodology, Eiser *et al.* (1992) asked mothers and fathers separately to rate the adjustment of their children. In this study, the children were being treated for one of five conditions; diabetes, asthma, cardiac disease, epilepsy or leukemia. Mothers and fathers were separately asked to rate the children's behaviour (using a version of the Child and Adolescent Adjustment Profile (Ellsworth 1979)). Factor analysis of this scale produced a satisfactory six factor solution. These sub-scales measured the following types of behaviour; frustration/hostility, (picked quarrels, been unable to accept difficulties); dependence, (asked unnecessary help), rule- following, (not responded to discipline), peer-relations, (invited others to play, tried to get along with others), work, (did work carefully, finished tasks) and withdrawal (sat and stared, appeared listless and apathetic). In addition, parents rated the extent to which the child was restricted by the disease. Ratings of restrictiveness were made on seven Likert-type scales, and referred to the extent to which the child was thought to be restricted in terms of school achievement, sports, ability to go out alone, age-appropriate independence, relationships with friends, relationships with teachers and self-care. Ratings of adjustment and restrictiveness differed between mothers and fathers. Children with leukemia or epilepsy were rated by their mothers as having more adjustment difficulties, especially on sub-scales measuring frustration/hostility. These groups were also perceived to experience most restrictions. Children with epilepsy or asthma were perceived to have greatest difficulties with respect to interactions with peers, and children with leukemia were rated as having most difficulties in relation to school and achievements. Mothers' ratings also suggested that they perceived greater adjustment difficulties among older children.

Fathers' ratings of their children's adjustment were not differentiated in relation to age, gender or disease group. However, there were some differences in their ratings of restrictions, with fathers of children with epilepsy rating their children to be specially restricted. These data raise some difficulties in interpreting information about childrens' adjustment which is based on one source of information only, as very different pictures emerge depending on whether mothers or fathers are used as informants. In addition, there were indications that ratings of adjustment were influenced by parents' perceptions of the child's restrictions. Children were rated as having more adjustment difficulties, especially on the subscales measuring peer-relations and work, as the restrictions associated with the disease increased.

Loneliness and social isolation

It is possible that the experience of chronic disease sets children apart from their healthy age-mates. Being aware that they have a life-long or chronic condition may make some feel more vulnerable but others respond by feeling special, or chosen in some way. The way in which children think about the condition and its consequences, as well as the length of time they are required to spend in adult company, may result in different processes of development and relationships with both children and adults. Perhaps also there is an underlying assumption that children with chronic disease can be spoilt by their parents and other well-meaning adults, with the result that they become the cause of some resentment among healthy children. There are implications, too, that healthy children may resent the extra care and attention that they perceive to be lavished on sick children, resulting in further animosity. It is sometimes observed that children with chronic diseases appear happiest in hospital where they are confident and known to many staff. Children with diabetes are sometimes suspected of provoking hypoglycemic attacks, in order that they can be admitted to hospital. Mothers of children with leukemia are sometimes surprised that their child seems to be less put out by readmission that expected, and attribute this to some positive rewards that the child experiences. A familiar hospital environment can give a child more independence and freedom than experienced in school, where adult attention is shared with 30 or so other children.

There has been a tendency to focus on rather negative implications of chronic disease for social development. Thus, researchers have been concerned to describe the extent to which children with chronic disease are lonely or socially isolated. It is possible to point to a handful of studies that support this position. Again, much work has focussed on the adverse consequences of childhood cancer. These children have been reported to be less socially competent (Deasy-Spinetta, Spinetta & Oxman 1988) and are teased, isolated and avoided by peers (Chesler, Paris & Barbarin 1986). In her review of the psychological consequences of diabetes, Johnson (1980) concluded that there was little indication of psychological maladjustment in childhood diabetes, except that these children were more likely to be socially isolated.

Children with chronic disease can be an obvious target for ridicule, particularly when they *look* different. Drugs used to treat cancers or renal disease can have the effect (usually temporarily) of making the child look fat and bloated, with negative consequences for games and physical activities. Children can think up many cruel nicknames for fat class-mates! It is often only one child who is the ring-leader, but the distress caused to the sick child can be immeasurable.

Chronic disease may have different consequences for social interaction depending on specifics of the condition and its limitations, as well as factors such as age or gender (La Greca 1990). She suggests that diseases which limit physical exercise, interrupt daily activities, or alter physical appearance, are likely to have relatively greater impact on social adjustment. Given the particular importance of physical activity and the development of strength and muscular coordination in boys compared with girls, it might also be expected that diseases which limit the attainment of these skills may have relatively worse implications for boys' social development.

With respect to age, Ungerer *et al.* (1988) found that the social consequences of rheumatoid arthritis increased for young adults with the condition compared with younger, particularly school-aged children. This was attributed to the fact that parents tend to be responsible for the arrangement of social lives of young children, and expect to organise activities and transport. This becomes less true as children grow older and more independent about where they go. Limited mobility becomes very much more of a problem for young adults as their peers are able to move around without parental help.

There are also many methodological problems inherent in much of the work reviewed so far. Ratings of loneliness or social isolation are often based on teacher reports. Teachers are invariably aware of the child's diagnosis, and their ratings may therefore reflect some stereo-typic beliefs about functioning in children with cancer as much as any characteristic of the child's behaviour. Teachers' perspectives reflect an important component of the child's behaviour in the classroom, but may not necessarily be shared by the children themselves. Yet very little work has been concerned with the status of the child with cancer in the classroom, as perceived by healthy peers.

An exception is a report by Noll *et al.* (1991) who studied the psy-chosocial adaptation of 24 children with cancer in the classroom both from their own and peer ratings of sociability, isolation and mutual friendships. Assessments of the child's tendencies to act in sociable, aggressive or isolated ways were made by the child with cancer and peers. Each child's popularity was assessed using an index of overall status within the peer group. In addition, a measure of mutual friend-ship was computed, and self-reported indices of social competence and self-worth were made by the child with cancer. The results support previous findings based on teachers' reports, in suggesting that children with cancer have a reputation for being socially isolated and withdrawn. However, findings from the sociometric data failed to show any differ-ences between healthy children and those with cancer in terms of their actual status within the peer group. Children with cancer were as popular as other children, though they tended to have slightly fewer reciprocated friends.

The focus on loneliness and social isolation very much masks the potentially more positive effects of chronic disease on social develop-ment. The experience of illness may provide children with the opportu-nity to develop more empathic responses to others, and act as an impetus for increases in awareness of others' feelings, responses and emotions. Certainly these arguments have been put forward with respect to the experience of more minor and everyday illness experiences (Parmelee 1986). Despite the hypothesised beneficial effects of chronic illness, little systematic investigation has been conducted. There is, instead, a num-ber of case reports and much autobiographical information to suggest that positive benefits of chronic disease can be identified. One of the earliest reports (Binger *et al.* 1969) described a child with cancer who was believed to be unaware of the diagnosis. Discussions with the child showed that he was so tuned in to others' feelings that he did not raise the topic despite his own concern because he was aware of the distress it might cause. The extent to which children with chronic disease are able to develop heightened empathy and concern for others, or the extent to which this is in any way a generalised response, is not clear. Clinicians often note that a relatively high proportion of survivors of childhood disease go into the caring professions, but again this has not been confirmed empirically. There is, however, some related evidence to suggest that healthy siblings who are exposed to chronic childhood disease in the family are more considerate than age-matched controls who have not had this experience (cf. Horwitz & Kazak 1988) (see Chapter 9).

The importance of this area of work is not merely academic, but needs to be considered in relation to work with healthy children, and theoretical assumptions about the role of childhood friendships for adjustment throughout adolescence and adult life. Peer relationships during childhood are considered to be fundamental to the development of adequate social skills and the attainment of a healthy self-concept (Hartup 1983). As increasing numbers of children with chronic disease survive into adulthood, it is important to ensure that any adverse social consequences are minimized. To this end, more systematic and methodologically sound research concerned with social consequences for children are necessary. Beyond this, it is also imperative to consider the social consequences for those who do survive to adult life; a question that is only recently becoming possible to ask, as the prognosis for many chronic conditions improves.

The way forward

Work in this area has traditionally centred on describing general behaviours in the classroom; that is, the concern whether children with chronic disease tend to have lower achievements than others, fewer friends or be less well- adjusted. Theoretically, it now seems important to identify ways in which children cope with specific incidents in school, rather than attempt to describe ways in which they generally respond (Quittner 1992). Within this tradition, methods involve describing problem situations to children, or using short video vignettes. Children are asked if they have ever experienced such situations, and exactly what they did to cope with the situation (Wallander & Hardy 1991).

A related procedure involves tracking the child's response to naturally occurring stressors, including the transition from junior to high school, or school entry itself. How do children's experiences in confronting and managing the demands of a chronic disease carry over to determine how they cope with more routine developmental stressors? Studying coping in children with chronic disease has implications for understanding the development of long-term coping and resourcefulness.

At a practical level, medical staff are keen to emphasise that chronic disease does not inevitably jeopardise the potential attainment of a 'normal life', but parents themselves often complain that conflicting advice is given about how best to achieve this. On the one hand, children should take part in all the games and activities enjoyed by other children, on the other, they may look different from everyone else, be restricted physically, or need to keep away from other children to reduce the risk of contracting a contagious disease. Treatment demands the need to take medication or undergo physiotherapy during the school day which makes it quite clear that the child is not 100 per cent normal. In addition, regular hospital appointments are the norm. Even in a condition such as leukemia, where treatment ceases after a defined period (usually two years), children are still required to return for check-ups almost indefinitely. Parents feel cheated that they were led to believe that life would return to normal when treatment ends, but in fact, this does not happen.

Improved hospital–school liaison could go some way to increase the child's chances to attain a 'normal life'. It has consistently been shown that stereotyping and lack of knowledge and understanding, characterises many adults' views about chronic childhood disease. There is room for much health education, directed at teachers and healthy children, which is essential for good integration in the classroom. Hospitals have an obligation to provide formal and systematic education in schools, especially when a child is diagnosed. However, support should not be restricted to the period around the diagnosis. On-going support may also be necessary, and further help during times of particular crisis. Teachers may feel specially unable to cope when a child dies. Their ability to deal with children's confusion and grief may be hampered by their own personal grief and inexperience with death.

Although children with chronic disease face some difficulties in the school environment, these are frequently less than those which confront individuals moving to the less protected adult world of work and independent living. In the next chapter, I would like to consider the difficulties faced by adolescents with chronic disease as they struggle to attain a balance between the imposed dependence of the condition, and achievement of desired independence and autonomy.

CHAPTER 4

'Storm and Stress'
The Impact of Chronic Disease During Adolescence

The developmental tasks of adolescence

Chronic disease has a unique impact during adolescence. During this time, families face many changes in their relationships both with the child and with each other. Demands for autonomy need to be recognised, and accommodated within the family environment. Adolescents begin to question parents' norms and values (Elkind 1967), and require more involved reasoning and explanations as justification of adult sanctions (Baumrind 1978). Mother–son relationships appear to be particularly vulnerable during this period (Hill 1987; Steinberg 1985).

The challenge of adolescence is to achieve the desired independence and autonomy, while at the same time, maintaining close and supportive ties with the nuclear family. These achievements cannot be made while adolescents continue to adopt child-like attachments to parents; neither can they be successful if ties are irreversibly broken. Becoming an autonomous individual and maintaining an interdependent relationship with one's parents are not mutually exclusive. They are complementary behaviours and part of normal family growth and development during adolescence.

The process of separation–individuation can be construed as a continuum. At one end, normal adjustment is achieved where adolescents develop their own identity while remaining connected to the family as an independent member. At the other end of the continuum, a process of alienation can be observed, characterized by disruptive behaviour, rejection of cultural and family values, and potential suicide. Many sociologists argue that the combination of cognitive and psychological changes that occur during adolescence, coupled with contemporary social changes across generations, make this period one of particular difficulty for adolescents and their families (Simmons & Blyth 1987). Traditionally, adolescence has been characterized as a period of 'storm and stress'; a time when individuals rebel against adult authority and question conventional norms and sanctions (Hall 1904).

Adolescence can be a particularly stressful time for parents. Pasley and Gecas (1984) found that 62 per cent of mothers and 64 per cent of fathers reported it to be the most difficult stage of parenting. Parents reported difficulties relating to their loss of control over the adolescent and fear for the adolescent's safety because of increased independence. Parents also reported that they were annoyed by the adolescent's behaviour. Loud music, unruly dress, outrageous hair-cuts all characterise adolescents, and all irritate parents and society more generally. Similar conclusions were reached by Small, Cornelius and Eastman (1983). Parents reported difficulties relating to the adolescent's demand for autonomy, failure to follow parental advice and deviant behaviour. The increased aggravation relating to adolescent behaviour can have negative implications for parents' marital relationships, (Rollins & Feldman 1970) and life satisfaction more generally (Hoffman & Manis 1978).

Adolescent difficulties are expected by, and sometimes encouraged within our culture. One 14-year-old boy described himself as follows: 'I'm a teenager; it's my job to be difficult!'

How chronic disease can compromise the attainment of developmental tasks
In the past, there was little attempt to document the specific difficulties of adolescents with chronic disease, largely because of the limited life expectancy associated with many conditions which precluded the possibility of long-term survival. Thus, it has only recently been acknowledged that adolescents with chronic disease face very special difficulties in their attempts to attain independence and autonomy. Successful separation from the nuclear family, career choices, marriage and parenting are difficult for all adolescents and young adults, but especially so for those with chronic disease.

The occurrence of chronic disease during adolescence is likely to exaggerate further the challenges of the adolescent period. At a time when peers are rapidly establishing their own independence and autonomy, the adolescent with chronic disease may meet many obstacles. Some may stem from a very real dependence on parents for help in administering treatment. Newly diagnosed patients for example, may be forced to rely on parents for help while they learn to implement procedures themselves, and even long-established patients may depend on parents during crisis periods, or even for routine treatments that they are unable to administer alone. Patients with cystic fibrosis, for example, sometimes remain dependent on parents for daily physiotherapy and are never able to manage this aspect of the treatment completely alone. Even when adolescents are proficient in most aspects of self-care, they may be forced to rely on parents for transport to hospital appointments, help in communicating with medical staff, or practical assistance with treatment at specific times, particularly during acute illness. While some degree of dependence may be unavoidable, the adolescent is particularly likely to resent dependence that is imposed by parents, i.e. where parental anxiety about the disease becomes so intense that they impose restrictions that are perceived by the adolescent to be unnecessary and fussy. In many different ways, chronic disease is likely to challenge developing autonomy particularly during this period.

Employment and future prospects
Further challenges occur in relation to future expectations and plans. Certain careers are difficult to pursue. For example, patients with diabetes or epilepsy may meet some obstacles. They tend only to be offered sedentary work in the armed or police forces (Tattersall & Jackson 1982); other restrictions may be imposed where the work involves heavy or dangerous machinery. Hicks and Hicks (1991) reported that 'potential safety hazard' was the most frequent reason given by companies for not employing individuals with epilepsy. Teta *et al.* (1986) also found that survivors of child and adolescent cancer faced rejection from the armed services and college and had difficulty obtaining health and life insurances. Job discrimination was reported by 20 per cent (Wasserman *et al.* 1987), 42 per cent (Fobair *et al.* 1986) and 54 per cent (Feldman 1980) of long-term survivors of childhood cancer.

Exclusion from the armed forces was felt to have a long-lasting effect by some men, since they were consequently excluded from access to this form of further training. Green, Zevon and Hall (1991) found that unemployment among male survivors of childhood cancer did not differ from population norms, but was above average for female survivors. While there may be little real reason why individuals should not pursue any career they wish regardless of their disease, they are likely to meet more hidden prejudices amongst employees, who fear increases in days absence, benefit costs, and distress among other workers. Current legislation appears to have been relatively successful in that employees are now more prepared to consider workers regardless of their health status, but attitudes remain slow to change (Hicks & Hicks 1991).

Even for those with diabetes, (frequently considered to be one of the least restricting of chronic conditions), there are risks of unemployment for some (Robinson *et al.* 1989a) and somewhat limited employment opportunities for others (Robinson *et al.* 1989b). In this latter study, just 1 per cent of firms said they would not consider an individual with diabetes for employment. Other firms anticipated difficulties where the work was strenuous, or involved working at heights, alone, with dangerous machinery, travelling, or shift work and irregular hours. Confronted by some of these objections, adolescents with diabetes may well feel that their career opportunities are restricted. In the related study reported by Robinson (1989a), evidence that the restrictions are real was apparent in that unemployment rates among those with diabetes were higher (22% for females and 8% for males) compared with a matched control group (12% for females and 5% for males).

Aside from the real restrictions that may be encountered in terms of employment opportunities, adolescents with chronic disease may harbour more emotional concerns with regard to their personal lives. Female patients particularly tend to be concerned about their physical attractiveness, marriage eligibility, and ability to have children. Especially for those with certain diseases, such as diabetes, these concerns are very real; pregnancy being associated with unique problems for mothers with diabetes.

Compliance with medical advice and treatment

Clinically, there is no doubt that adolescents are often perceived to be rather troublesome and noncompliant patients, especially compared with younger children (Smith et al. 1979; Jacobson et al. 1987; Lemanek 1991). Clinic attendance may become erratic or cease altogether. There may be a decline in compliance with medical advice and treatments, and increase in challenges to adult authority. These difficult behaviours are generally explained within a 'storm and stress' view of adolescence; that is, non compliance with medical advice is seen to parallel more general rebellion and disagreements with parents. This view is limited partly by empirical evidence that adolescence is not inevitably a time of such undue strife, and many adolescents do maintain warm and close relationships with their parents. Second, there has been no evidence that adolescents who have most difficulty in adherence are also those who score high on measures of rebellion or risk-taking. Third, noncompliance occurs more frequently in some conditions compared with others (La Greca 1990a).

'The most consistent links between adolescence and poor adherence have been obtained for chronic diseases with complex treatment regimens, such as diabetes and asthma, or for regimens that affect physical appearance. In contrast, Phipps and DeCuir- Whalley (1991) found adolescents to be more adherent than younger children with a regimen for bone-marrow transplantation that involved aversive medications' (La Greca 1990a, p.430).

Phipps and DeCuir-Whalley (1990) speculated that in situations where control is so totally stripped from adolescents, as is involved in procedures such as bone-marrow transplantation, depression and withdrawal may result in apathy and apparent compliance. The treatment may also have the effect of increasing dependency and regressive behaviour. Very sick adolescents have little energy to resist adult pressure, and therefore go along with medical advice. In contrast, younger children undergoing bone-marrow transplantation were more openly hostile and resistant to medications. This study questions the long-held view of a linear relationship between chronological age and noncompliance. Future work needs to consider more carefully the relationship between patients' efforts to comply and the demands of the treatment and extent of self-care involved. A confounding factor in the study by Phipps and DeCuir-Whalley (1990) may be that ratings of compliance were made by medical staff. The possibility that staff may judge adolescents' behaviour against an expectation that this group are necessarily noncompliant would result in more normative ratings. In contrast, staff may expect younger children to be cooperative and be surprised by their resistance. In terms of staff expectations, the result is that younger children are perceived to be less compliant than expected, and adolescents more so.

In addition, there is an increasing awareness that some of these apparently non-compliant and difficult behaviours are a result of physiological and hormonal changes that are part of adolescent development, rather than frankly disagreeable behaviour (Litt & Cuskey 1980). For example, puberty is associated with a marked decrease in insulin sensitivity, which complicates self-care in adolescents with diabetes (Bloch, Clemmons & Sperling 1987). The result, however, is that the adolescent may be blamed for the resulting poor health. Physicians become exasperated, and a vicious cycle of mutual misunderstanding and distrust follows. Current work raises questions about the extent to which adolescents are deliberately less compliant than younger children. The processes linking an individual's perception of control over treatment with compliance is complex, and perhaps age dependent, with older children being more compliant where they perceive greater control. Understanding why chronic disease is uniquely challenging during adolescence is a question of major theoretical and practical importance.

Beliefs about disease and death

Elkind (1967) has described adolescence as a period of 'egocentrism'. The hall-mark of adolescent cognitive development is the ability 'to think about thinking', both their own and that of others. The emergence and awareness of this ability creates some difficulties, in that adolescents may fail to differentiate between the objects about which others are thinking and those that are central to their own thoughts. Coupled with adolescents' preoccupation with themselves, their appearance and their own behaviour, a logical error occurs, so that adolescents become convinced that they themselves are of central interest and concern to others.

This egocentric confusion has two consequences. First, adolescents create an *imaginary audience*. They believe that everyone is looking at them and are constantly concerned with how they appear to others. The audience is imaginary to the extent that others are rarely as pre-occupied with the adolescent as is believed, but the result may be a painful self-consciousness coupled with a search for escape and privacy. Although the belief in the imaginary audience usually disappears by late adolescence, a second confusion – the *personal fable*, lasts much longer. According to Elkind (1967), adolescents believe that their own thoughts and actions are original, new and special; unique and more intense than the experiences of others or previous generations. This belief in personal uniqueness colors adolescents' approach to life, resulting in a conviction of personal invulnerability and preparedness to take much greater risks than during any other period.

The concern with personal appearance is common to all adolescents, and many experience dissatisfaction with their looks and body shape. Chronic disease can aggravate the concern, especially in conditions associated with delayed physical maturity. Adolescents with cystic fibrosis, for example, are often dissatisfied with their appearance, sometimes going to extreme lengths to disguise and conceal those aspects which cause them most personal concern (Boyle *et al.* 1976). Similar concerns about physical immaturity appear to dominate the thoughts of girls suffering from Turner's syndrome. These girls are short and sterile and frequently need hormone treatment to reach physical maturity. Associated deficits in spatial and memory tasks and difficulties in distinguishing between facial expressions all contribute to frequent problems in social relationships (McCauley *et al.* 1987). In other conditions, especially cancer or renal disease, changes in body shape and appearance are more directly attributable to medical treatment. Regardless of the specific cause, the end result can be a pathological concern and anxiety about the individuals' body and general appearance. This may parallel the concerns of all adolescents, but takes on a new meaning among those with chronic disease.

The belief in a personal fable can have more damaging consequences, in that adolescents may be reluctant to accept the knowledge that they have a life-long or potentially fatal disease. With this reluctance goes a denial of the consequences of the disease, and refusal to acknowledge the importance of self-care and adherence to treatment. The poor compliance which is often noted in adolescents is perhaps related to the belief in a personal fable, or refusal to acknowledge personal vulnerability. Just as the normal adolescent may be reluctant to acknowledge the long-term risks associated with smoking, alcohol or drug-abuse, so those with diabetes find it hard to accept the possibility of long-term damage which may be associated with poor adherence and haemoglobin control.

Cognitive development during adolescence enables the individual to comprehend the nature and implications of the disease from a more scientific or medical perspective. Knowledge of biology and physiology means that the adolescent is able to acquire a more thorough understanding of the condition, and given the demands of self-care, many doctors and parents encourage this. Yet with such knowledge goes an insight into the potential complications of treatments and awareness of personal vulnerability. Greater knowledge can be accompanied by greater anxiety (Allen *et al.* 1984). While adolescents may develop the cognitive capacity to understand disease, they are often less well-prepared to handle the emotional consequences.

Expectations of autonomy

Chronic disease may challenge adolescents' move toward autonomy by increasing dependence on parents and medical staff. Parents may find it particularly difficult to allow adolescents as much freedom as other parents allow healthy adolescents, given their increased concern and anxiety about their child's health, and greater involvement in treatment regimens and hospital appointments. There is a frequent assumption among health professionals that chronic disease will inevitably create conflict between adolescents and their parents over issues of independence and desires to move away from parental authority. Despite this wide-spread assumption, very little empirical work has been concerned to establish its validity. In an early study by Partridge *et al.* (1972), adolescents and children with diabetes were reported not to differ from healthy peers in terms of the ages when they expected to be themselves responsible for a number of different tasks, such as deciding on their own hair-style and dress, or the time they should be home at night.

Autonomous behaviours can be considered in two categories; the first including those which are specific to the management of disease, and the second including those which are more general and relevant to all individuals. In the first category, the question is when children or adolescents with diabetes should themselves be responsible for their own insulin injections or blood-testing; for those with cystic fibrosis with when they should manage their own physiotherapy. In the second category, the concern is with everyday independence; when should adolescents make their own decisions about where they go, how late they stay out at night, or whom they are with? More importantly, to what extent should these decisions be compromised because the child has a chronic condition?

Disease-related activities

With regard to when adolescents should be responsible for their own self-care, most work has focussed on those with diabetes. Johnson *et al.* (1982) argued that many children and adolescents were poorly informed about many details of self-care. Many knew so little about management of the disease that they could not realistically be expected to cope alone. They further hypothesised that there may be specific ages when management tasks are best taught. Thus, it was suggested that practical knowledge about diet and insulin reactions might be emphasised from about 6 years of age; self-injection could be taught at about 9 years, and urine testing from 12 years onwards. This should not be treated as a rigid framework, however, as it was clear that some children were able to understand complex information about the treatment at relatively younger age-levels.

Although some guide-lines have subsequently been published about when it is advisable for children to be responsible for aspects of their own treatment regimens, these have generally been based on general theories of child development, committee decisions and clinical judgment rather than empirical data. The issue is not purely academic, since inappropriate expectations about personal responsibility for treatment have sometimes been associated with poorer health status (Ingersoll *et al.* 1986). Expectations that either encourage independence before a child is ready, or undermine a child's ability with regard to self-care, can compromise compliance and the acquisition of related skills.

'Prescription of autonomy in self-care before the child is developmentally or cognitively capable of mastering a skill may result in failure to achieve goals and discourage future initiative. Conversely, expectations that are substantially below the child's actual capabilities could inhibit the achievement of autonomy by promoting excessive dependence on others or lead to the assertion of independence in other, less desirable ways. Thus, selection of developmentally appropriate diabetes education and treatment goals could improve diabetic control and adjustment to the disease'. (Wysocki *et al.* in press)

Wysocki *et al.* (1990) surveyed 229 health professionals about the ages at which they expected children to master 38 different diabetes-related skills. It was anticipated that all the tasks included could be mastered by children 14 years of age or less. Children were expected to be able to report hypoglycemia at the youngest ages (6.5 years), but to be unable to master other tasks (for example, stating indications for insulin dose change and planning exercise routines considering insulin schedule and diet, till much later (about 14 years). There was, however, considerable variability in responses, indicating little broad agreement between professionals. In addition, physicians expected later mastery of a number of skills compared with nursing staff or psychologists, raising the issue that different members of the health care team may give different advice.

In a related study, Wysocki *et al.* (in press) surveyed 490 parents of adolescents with diabetes about the ages at which the felt their children were *capable* of self-care with respect to different aspects of diabetes management. Parents were encouraged to think in terms of ability, rather than in terms of compliance and whether or not their adolescent actually did these tasks. These data were also compared with the estimates made by medical staff reported in the earlier paper (Wysocki *et al.* 1990). For 33 of the 38 skills assessed, median mastery ages estimated by medical staff exceeded those made by parents by one year or more. Thus, for many items, parents reported earlier skill mastery than expected by professionals. These skills consisted largely of those involving rote or motor acts (for example, using a lancet to obtain an adequate blood sample), or those in which the consequences of an error were immediate and aversive (for example, treating hypoglycemia; anticipating and preventing hypoglycemia). In contrast, parents reported attainment of other skills consistently above the ages anticipated by medical staff. These skills were characterised by extensive reliance on planning and anticipation (for example, anticipating and preventing hyperglycemia; adjust insulin dose); or involved tasks which are infrequently required of adolescents (for example, completing urine ketone tests), and those where the consequences of errors are not immediately apparent or only loosely related together (for example, using meal plan in restaurants).

The results of these studies together suggest that substantial differences exist between professionals and parents in their perceptions of adolescents' abilities to be responsible for their own self-care. Such discrepancies may contribute to communication difficulties between families and professionals. At the same time, it is important to remember that the data refer to perceptions of tasks which adolescents might be expected to manage themselves, and not to whether they actually perform such activities. Neither are the data relevant to the issue of whether or not it is appropriate for adolescents to be responsible for tasks that are within their ability levels. It may be that absolute responsibility for self management tasks should be deferred for some time beyond when individuals are theoretically able to master any given skill.

While some children and adolescents may clamour to be responsible for their own care, others assume responsibility more reluctantly. Much failure in treatment implementation appears to stem from a lack of agreement and communication between patients and their parents as to whom is responsible for day-to-day management. Anderson *et al.* (1991)

relate the extent of disagreements between mothers and their children with diabetes over responsibility for treatment to the child's haemoglobin control. Thus, the greater the disagreement, the worse the child's haemoglobin level. Problems arise where mother or child assumes that the other is responsible, but neither have clarified their roles or expectations about each other. Difficulties result from a failure to specify changes in responsibility for treatment as the adolescent matures.

The focus on diabetes in this context can be attributed to the degree to which treatment of diabetes is dependent on the acquisition of a number of self-care skills. Medical staff stress that long-term health is very much the personal responsibility of the patient. Few other conditions are associated with a need for such extensive personal care, although an element of patient responsibility is characteristic of many conditions.

One of the most common chronic diseases is asthma, and some consideration has been given to the issue of patient self-care management and its implications in this context. McNabb, Wilson-Pessano and Jacobs (1986) emphasise that good self-management goes far beyond simply taking prescribed medication. Children can engage in behaviours which precipitate attacks, or aggravate the severity of an attack. For example, children can understand that they are allergic to animals, but still insist on having a family pet. They can know that they are aggravated by grasses and pollen, but decide to take the risk as everyone else is playing football.

They can also engage in a variety of other behaviours which serve to limit or reduce the likelihood of experiencing an asthma attack. Such behaviours include:

- *Prevention;* those that serve to avoid an attack or prevent the occurrence of symptoms, such as avoiding allergens, keeping medication accessible or developing some form of mental imagery to reduce the likelihood of an attack;

- *Intervention;* removing oneself from exposure to a precipitating agent; remaining calm during an attack, or practicing some intervention strategy;

- *Compensation;* accepting responsibility for self-care; discussing the condition with peers; cooperating with necessary treatments and avoiding manipulative behaviours;

- *Managing external factors;* particularly authority figures who obstruct the child's self-management and learning to cope with family difficulties that are known to precipitate attacks.

Non-disease related activities

With regard to the question of autonomy in relation to non disease-related activities, Seagull and Somers (1991) contacted 192 adolescents, including 96 with a chronic disease, and their parents, to establish any differences between those with chronic disease and a healthy population in terms of the age when they expected to exhibit various autonomous behaviours. The chronically sick group included those with diabetes (39), asthma (17), and a number of other conditions (not specified). As reported previously for the general population (Feldman & Quatman 1988), parents held significantly later expectations than adolescents, i.e. they anticipated that adolescents would be responsible for their own self-care and activities later than was expected by adolescents themselves. In addition, fathers held later autonomy expectations than mothers. There were no differences in expectations as a function of gender. Neither were there differences between the healthy adolescents and those with chronic disease, except with regard to health behaviours. Compared with the chronically sick group, healthy adolescents had later expectations in relation to smoking behaviour, being responsible for making their own doctor or dentist appointments, taking medication, and sleeping the night at a friend's house. They had younger expectations with regard to staying home alone when ill, going to the doctor without an adult, and changing from pediatric to adult care. Some of these results are quite surprising. For example, why should adolescents with chronic disease report that they expect to start smoking when younger than the healthy group? Smoking creates special difficulties for those with respiratory diseases such as asthma over and above the normal health hazards.

Some of the other findings suggest that adolescents with chronic disease do see themselves to be highly dependent on medical care. They have later expectations regarding staying home alone when ill, or going to the doctor without an adult, despite the fact that they must have far greater experience of going to the doctor. However, the real thrust of the findings lie in the lack of differences between the groups in non-illness related areas assessed. Families of those with chronic disease were not more protective toward their adolescents than other families. This issue merits further attention, especially since the response rate in this study was very low (25.7%). Perhaps those who declined to take part did so because they did not want to acknowledge an issue which was recognized to be a source of underlying conflict.

Yet autonomy should not necessarily be defined so narrowly in terms of relationships between chronological age and the attainment of different self-care behaviours. Chronic disease may undermine adolescents' confidence to implement self-care tasks as well as their social skills in more general contexts. Differences between chronically sick and healthy groups on variables such as self-esteem, self-confidence and efficacy have been pursued in a number of studies. Although often based on heterogeneous populations including younger children and adolescents, there is some support for the notion that chronic diseases generally compromise the attainment of autonomy as measured by these concepts. Havermans and Eiser (1991) found that children with diabetes endorsed stronger internal locus of control beliefs than healthy children, perhaps rejecting the fact that they acknowledged the role of their own behaviour in promoting good health. However, they scored lower than healthy children on a measure of self-efficacy, suggesting that they felt less confident or able to implement these health related behaviours. Thus, although those with diabetes recognised the potential importance of their own behaviour for health, they were less confident in their abilities to implement these tasks. This finding may be especially relevant in planning intervention programmes, suggesting that the emphasis may need to be as much on bolstering children's and adolescents' confidence to perform self-care as any direct teaching about what should be done.

The influence of peers

Adolescence is often described as a period in which peer influence increases at the expense of parental authority. Furthermore, the influence of peers is often viewed as negative. This assertion stems largely from research concerned with smoking, alcohol or drug-taking behaviour, in which it has been observed that adolescents who participate in these activities tend to have friends who also smoke, drink or take drugs. The 'peer-group pressure' hypothesis rests on the assumption that adolescents' use of legal or illegal drugs is predictable from the drug-taking behaviour of peers (Strickland & Pittman 1984).

The peer-group pressure hypothesis has also been used to explain peer influences on self care behaviour among chronically sick children. Again, the influence may often be very largely negative. This may be attributable to the behaviour of the sick child, and stem from a desire to inform as few people as possible. Where peers understand very little, or nothing, about the disease, they can hardly be blamed for not helping. Peers can be an obstruction to good management, simply because they fail to understand the requirements of good treatment. They can also be more destructive, in that they understand the requirements of the treatment, but encourage non-adherence. It is sometimes difficult for the adolescent to comply satisfactorily with treatment advice when in the company of friends. For example, girls with diabetes may understand very well the need for regular food intake, but have difficulty eating at frequent intervals as friends are always dieting or eating junk food. Peers become increasingly influential in determining choice of foods and frequency of consumption during adolescence.

Much research work seems to be based on the assumption that parents necessarily provide positive support to their child in implementing treatment tasks, while peers provide at best erratic support, and at worst, obstacles to successful implementation. The empirical literature which is developing in this area provides little support for such assumptions. Rather, parents and peers provide different kinds of support depending on the situation. McNabb, Wilson-Pessano and Jacobs (1986) provided clear evidence that adults, including parents and teachers, could sometimes prevent the child with asthma from taking appropriate self-care action. In contrast, friends could be highly supportive. In a study involving adolescents with diabetes (aged 10–14 years), La Greca (1990b) reported that although peers were generally less supportive than parents and other family members, they were more effective in providing particular kinds of support. Peers were especially helpful in making adjustments to their own meal-times and exercise schedules in order to accommodate the diabetic regimen. They were also more likely to provide 'emotional support'; being available to discuss the implications of diabetes. It is likely that during adolescence, patients with diabetes begin to feel more comfortable in discussing some aspects of the disease with friends rather than parents. These issues may centre on concerns about the future, especially in relation to sexual behaviour, or the consequences of drug-taking or smoking.

It is now recognised that the 'peer-group pressure' hypothesis is overly simplistic (Eiser et al. 1991) friendships are based on multiple dimensions of similarity and not simply on smoking behaviour. The question of why some children choose friends who are sympathetic and helpful while others choose friends who are less supportive, may be more crucial for future work.

Use of health care services

The diagnosis of chronic disease in a child is associated with many changes in everyday family life and experiences, including the very real demands, both practical and emotional, necessitated by regular clinic attendance. Out-patient attendance is always time-consuming, and particularly so for families who live in rural areas, have little access to public transport, or do not own a car. Specialist clinics are often held in large hospitals in the centre of the city, and this may mean that driving, and finding a parking place for a private car is difficult and expensive. Even so, most parents prefer to drive themselves if possible, since there are even more difficulties to be encountered on public transport. For example, children with leukemia may undergo anesthetisation when experiencing lumbar punctures. As the effects of anesthetisation lessen, the child may experience bouts of vomiting. Anxiety that trains will be late and children begin vomiting before they reach home deters many parents from using public transport.

Emotionally, parents tend to report heightened anxiety immediately before clinic attendance (McCarthy 1975), and this applies especially to conditions characterised by periods of illness and remission, such as leukemia and juvenile arthritis. One or other parent may need to take time off work to accompany the sick child. While parents in some countries are legally allowed time off work when their child has a serious illness, this is not a routine entitlement in the U.K. Arrangements need to be made for younger children at home during the day, or for older children after school.

Yet appropriate care of chronically sick children is dependent on regular clinic attendance and careful monitoring of disease progression. The child's health is critically dependent on clinic attendance, and by implication, the development of a close, trusting relationship between doctor and patient. It is one of parents' most frequent complaints that they rarely see the same doctor on two successive clinic visits. For children with chronic disease and their parents, it is essential to provide an acceptable clinic service. It may not be possible to provide a service which patients positively enjoy attending, but it should be possible to provide one which patients perceive to be professional, competent and sympathetic.

From this point of view, good information about parents' satisfaction with services is vital to achieve effective changes in practice and go some way toward maximising parent cooperation and involvement in the care of their child. Charlop et al. (1987) noted that the evaluation of clinic activities can provide a 'self-corrective' feed-back mechanism which is essential in the development of services. With regard to satisfaction with care among adult patients, two major dimensions have been identified. These include accessibility or convenience of care, and physician conduct (Doyle & Ware 1977; Lebow 1983).

As in adult work, communication between physician, parent and child is important, although perhaps more problematic. Pantell et al. (1982) showed that doctors tend to direct their remarks to parents rather than children, even where the child has a chronic condition and has been seeing the same physician for several years. Where doctors did talk to children, they tended to ask questions about symptoms, but direct information about treatment and follow-up appointments to parents.

It is unclear the extent to which studies concerned with adult patients, or children receiving general pediatric care is directly extrapolatable to those with special health care needs (Krahn, Eisert & Fifield 1990). Children with chronic or handicapping conditions frequently attend specialist centres and are required to have extensive interaction with health care teams, rather than specific individuals. Contact with different specialists has frequently been noted as an additional source of discontent among parents of children with chronic disease. It is unfortunate that much work concerned with the evaluation of services tends to be rather parochial in nature. One of the first steps toward correcting this bias may be in the development of assessment instruments which are applicable across a range of settings.

Krahn, Eisert and Fifield (1990) produced a ten-item questionnaire for use with populations of chronic and handicapping disorders. Factor analyses of parents' ratings produced a four-factor solution, including items to assess *general satisfaction* (quality and kind of service, preparedness to recommend to others or return themselves); *clarity of communication* (clarity and accuracy of communication, complexity of paperwork); *pre-appointment wait and information* (length of time waiting for initial appointment) and *efficiency* (total length of appointment, punctuality of staff). In addition to these questionnaire-based responses, parents were encouraged to make additional comments themselves. These indicated that convenience and accessibility were important additional determinants of satisfaction with care, as previously reported for adult patients (Lebow 1983).

Whenever assessments of satisfaction with care have been made among children with chronic disease and their parents, similar conclusions have been reached as with adult patients; i.e. physician communication skills, impressions of competence and efficiency are important. In studies of young adolescents with diabetes, Weinberger, Cohen and Mazzuca (1984) found that staff attitudes (but not knowledge) were predictive of patients' metabolic control. Patients were in better control where staff worked together as a health care team. Bloomfield and Farquhar (1990) similarly found that metabolic control and number of emergency hospital admissions were improved when children attended specialist rather than general pediatric clinics. The implications from both these studies might be that certain attributes of clinics, particularly organization and staff approaches to patients, may influence childrens' attitudes to the disease and willingness to adhere to medical advice, resulting in changes in haemoglobin levels.

More direct evidence on this issue is provided in a study by Hanson, Hengeller and Burghen (1987). Ninety-six adolescents with diabetes and their parents were questioned about their satisfaction with the health care provided. Satisfaction was assessed from ratings of the physician's personal qualities, professional competence and cost and convenience of care. All family members tended to rate the physician's personal qualities and competence positively, but held more negative attitudes to cost and convenience of care. Adolescents' perceptions of the competence of the physician was associated with better metabolic control. Adherence to treatment was positively associated with fathers' attitudes to staff competence, but only marginally associated with mothers' and adolescents' perceptions of competence. Nevertheless, these results indicate that perceptions of clinic organization and staff competence can influence patient adherence to treatment, and consequently metabolic control, (though it is possible that patients who were in good control had more positive interactions with physicians, were praised for their good adherence behaviours, and therefore perceive the whole medical encounter to be more successful and enjoyable than patients who were in less good control.)

Transition from pediatric to adult-based services
Particular difficulties for children with chronic disease and their families can often arise during adolescence. While there may be many factors contributing to these difficulties, an additional problem can sometimes be attributable to the need to transfer from the pediatric to the adult clinics. For some children, who have attended the same pediatric clinic for much of their lives, the transition can be particularly threatening, and many patients may be tempted to put off the date of transfer as long as possible. It can happen, for example, that survivors of childhood cancer are still being seen at follow-up pediatric clinics, even well into their thirties!

Childrens' hospitals tend to care for children up to age 16 or 18 years, although many exceptions occur. In 1938, the American Academy of Pediatrics noted that this was indeed so. By 1972, however, these recommendations were changed to suggest that childrens' hospitals should provide services for those up to 21 years of age. The void in services for patients with long-term or chronic conditions was recognised.

'There are special circumstances (e.g. a chronic illness or disability) in which, if mutually agreeable to the pediatrician, the patient, and, when appropriate, the patient's family, the services of the pediatrician may continue to be the optimal source of care past the age of 21 years' (Editorial, *Pediatrics* 1972, p.463).

Special problems arise for those with life-threatening conditions such as cancer or cystic fibrosis, since in these cases doctors need to consider the patient's potential life- expectancy. It is often felt to be inappropriate to put patients through any inconvenience relating to changes in clinic if anticipated life-expectancy is seriously compromised. For most patients with chronic, but non life-threatening conditions, however, the question is not whether transfer should occur, but when. Decisions about when patients transfer are usually taken by the pediatrician, sometimes in collaboration with the family, and usually on the grounds of social or physical maturity of the child.

There are a number of potential barriers to successful transfer, (Schidlow & Fiel 1990). These have variously been attributed to attitudes of patients, the family, the pediatrician, or the adult physician. Patients may become excessively dependent on the pediatrician, particularly when the illness is long-standing. By the nature of the illness, some patients may be physically immature. (For example, growth and sexual development may be retarded in those with cystic fibrosis or cancer). They may also be emotionally immature and socially isolated, lacking the social support or emotional resources to enable them to deal effectively with any kind of change. Transfer may also coincide with periods of poor adherence and difficult behaviour, characteristic of some adolescents with chronic disease (Johnson 1988).

The family, too, may raise some objections. Many realize that control over the child's illness, and their own role in ensuring that treatments are adhered to, is in any case being eroded as the child matures, and fear that this will be exacerbated with the transfer to the adult clinic. Families may not necessarily share the medical view of the seriousness of their child's condition, and over- or under-estimate likely survival. Families may also have developed an over-dependency on staff in pediatric clinics, fostered by gratitude for their skill at diagnosis and care of the child during the initial worrying, and perhaps very frightening stages of the illness.

The pediatrician may feel particularly proud of some patients, and be reluctant to relinquish control, especially where patients have flourished and done well against all odds. The pediatrician may well feel reluctant to initiate any change in what is perceived to be a very satisfactory situation, and feel confident that adequate care can continue to be provided.

Finally, adult physicians may feel reluctant to accept patients from pediatric clinics, particularly where they feel they lack expertise to deal with what are traditionally diseases of children. This problem arises in the transfer of patients with conditions such as cystic fibrosis, which has traditionally been confined to childhood. It is less of a problem in conditions such as diabetes, where adult physicians have considerable experience and expertise.

The organisation of diabetes clinics can vary substantially. Some differences between pediatric and adult clinics have been attributed to the training and experience of the physicians themselves. Marteau and Baum (1984) found that adult physicians estimated significantly greater levels of diabetes related morbidity and mortality than pediatricians, and demanded stricter levels of blood-sugar control in their patients. Pediatricians were unlikely to have much experience of long-term complications in their patients, as these generally develop only after many years. This lack of experience led them to under-estimate the likely occurrence of complications in comparison with adult physicians, who spend much of their professional time dealing with diabetes-related complications. Other workers suggest that adult physicians tend to encourage greater independence and self-care, urging patients to communicate with them directly, rather than rely on parents to act as intermediaries (Cerreto & Travis 1984).

Although there may be many pit-falls in transferring from one clinic to another, it is inevitable that pediatric patients have to make the change at some point, and some may approach the experience more positively than others. There may be some advantages in attending an adult-orientated clinic without parents, especially if the young patient has concerns which could not easily be raised in the presence of parents. Many young patients may welcome the move to the adult clinic, and the opportunities to discuss issues of sexuality or drug-taking with the physician alone (Cerreto & Travis 1984).

Nevertheless, in recognition of the potential barriers to treatment during the adolescent and young adult age-group, a number of alternative types of clinic have been set up (Walsh 1985). During this period, patients may be offered one of four main types of service. These include continuation in the pediatric department or transfer directly to an adult clinic. One of the main concerns about the adult clinic is that patients may immediately come into contact with older patients who have experienced serious, often highly visible complications, such as blindness or amputations. There is a natural concern that younger patients may be disturbed by seeing individuals with visible signs of diabetes complications. This may make them feel very uncomfortable in the clinic and reduce or give up completely on attendance.

The alternatives are therefore clinics that cater more exclusively for young adult patients. In these settings, patients are less likely to meet others with serious complications. At the same time, they have the opportunity to meet with others of a similar age and perhaps share experiences and derive a degree of social support. In the third model for patient care, patients may therefore be offered a clinic organised by staff from the adult clinics but exclusively for a limited age-range. A fourth alternative is a joint service, where both the pediatrician and adult physician are in attendance. This has the advantage of allowing patients to be seen by the more familiar paediatrician until they feel comfortable to deal with the adult physician alone.

Salmi *et al.* (1986) followed 61 patients with diabetes for one year before and one year after their transfer from a pediatric clinic to a traditional adult clinic. The timing of the referral was made on the basis of physical maturity determined by the cessation of normal growth, full pubertal development and reasonable social maturation. The authors reported no significant deterioration in metabolic control on the first visit to the adult clinic, but some general improvement in control was noted during the first year in the adult clinic compared with levels achieved in the last year attending the pediatric clinic. Boys and patients with a shorter disease history appeared to cope more easily with the transition.

Eiser *et al.* (1992) studied 69 patients attending a clinic exclusively for patients under-25 years of age. Forty-one of these patients had been transferred from a pediatric clinic; the remainder having been diagnosed as young adults. Patients were asked to rate eight items (diet, exercise, school or work progress, family relations, avoidance of long-term complications, blood-glucose levels, insulin-testing and privacy) in terms of the importance assigned to them separately by staff in the pediatric and under-25 clinics. As predicted from the data reported by Marteau and Baum (1984), patients reported that pediatricians placed more emphasis on school progress and family relations compared with adult physicians, while adult physicians placed more emphasis on the importance of avoiding long-term complications, checking blood-sugar levels and exercising. Diet and insulin-testing were reported to be emphasised in both clinics, and patients' privacy was seen to be given little priority in either clinic.

Patients' informal comments confirmed that they find transferring clinics problematic:

> 'My first visit to the (adult) clinic really frightened me. The only reason for this was on this particular day while waiting to see the doctor, there appeared to be a large number of elderly patients with problems such as amputations, inability to walk very well, and very poor eye-sight. Although I realise that these are problems that can happen to a very badly diagnosed diabetic, I felt thoroughly depressed and hated my diabetes. Since that time I have got over my hatred, but still feel anxious coming to clinic.'

The mean age on transfer was 15.90 years (range=12–20 years). Patients were not routinely transferred on the grounds of physical maturity, but more likely for a number of social reasons. These included: to be with others of the same age 3, moving house 4, and the pediatric clinic was seen to be no longer suitable (usually not strict enough) 4, two patients transferred themselves, one wanted to use a different treatment which was not available in the pediatric clinic and one patient became pregnant. Generally, patients did not recall many difficulties for themselves, or their parents, resulting from the change-over of clinics. However, as also reported in the study by Salmi *et al.* (1986), women reported slightly more difficulties than men.

Eiser *et al.* concluded that patients recalled few difficulties about transferring from the pediatric clinic. For many patients, especially those who transferred clinics at the same time as they moved house, changed schools, or began work, the transfer seemed to proceed very smoothly. However, a minority of patients seemed to take the opportunity to opt out of hospital care altogether, and made no appearance in the under-25 clinic following their referral. While the transfer may therefore be relatively easy to manage for many patients, it needs to be remembered that such changes are likely to raise difficulties for some. It is particularly for these patients that care needs to be taken to ease the practical arrangements for transition, and that sources of potential conflict need to be minimized. Pediatricians and adult physicians need to be aware of some differences in their approach to patient care and education which may limit the acceptability of hospital-based care for some.

The issue of transfer of care from pediatric clinics has been discussed largely with reference to diabetes, since most empirical work has been conducted with this group. However, the issue is a general one, and of increasing concern as long-term survival in once fatal conditions of childhood, increase. Differences in approach between pediatricians and those who specialize in the treatment of adults can arise for children with cystic fibrosis, cancer, or renal disease, but have not yet been widely acknowledged.

An exception is work reported by Bywater (1981) and Cappelli, MacDonald and McGrath (1989), involving transfer of adolescents with cystic fibrosis from pediatric to adult based care. Bywater (1981) interviewed adolescents with cystic fibrosis, and reported that 52 per cent did not wish to be transferred to the adult clinic at a mandatory age of 16 years. Females were particularly anxious about the transfer, with 11 per cent of female patients stating that they would stop attending the hospital for treatment, if forced to attend the adult clinic. Both in relation to cystic fibrosis and diabetes, there is evidence that females find transfer more difficult. Bywater (1981) concluded that age in itself was not a valid indicator of patients' 'readiness' to transfer clinic. Other social and personality variables and gender, also seem important.

Cappelli *et al.* (1989) interviewed pediatric care-givers, adult care-givers, and three adult patients in an effort to determine their beliefs about the skills and knowledge necessary for successful transition to adult care. The interviews focussed on issues relating to medications, medical management and decision-making, physiotherapy, diet, exercise, parental involvement and knowledge of the disease. There was generally high agreement between pediatric and adult care-givers about the knowledge and skills essential to ensure satisfactory transfer. Based on these findings, a 'Readiness Questionnaire' was developed, including 15 knowledge items and 9 behaviour items. It was administered to 36 adolescents and young adults. In addition, all adolescents were rated by a care-giver on a four-point scale in terms of how well they were expected to handle the transition to adult care.

Adolescents' ratings on the Readiness Questionnaire and not chronological age related to caregivers' ratings of expected ability to transfer successfully. Cappelli *et al.* (1989) point to the limitations of using age as a marker for transfer, and suggest instead that care should be taken to ensure that adolescents are adequately prepared in terms of their knowledge and understanding of the disease.

Although this study suggests that pediatric and adult care-givers are agreed about the knowledge that is desirable for adult self-care, this does not imply that they necessarily convey information to patients in the same way, or indeed that patients may not perceive differences in the organisation of clinics, as was suggested in the research concerned with patients with diabetes. However, it would be useful to establish if pediatrians and adult physicians involved in the care of patients with diabetes agreed in theory about the information necessary for successful transition.

It may well be that any difficulties surrounding the transfer are experienced more by parents than the patient, and relate to parents' anxieties concerning their decreasing involvement in the implementation of treatment regimens. For parents, the transfer can be specially difficult to handle. They usually attend pediatric clinics regularly, and are well known there. They tend to ask the questions and report directly to staff about the child's health and behaviour. They are less welcome in adult clinics, and patients themselves are expected to report to staff. Attempts need to be made to help parents to accept their reduced role in patient management, which may often mean encouraging them to trust their child's judgment in relation to treatment adherence.

It is important to understand that the transfer from pediatric to adult-based care is but *one* of a number of transitions which are made during the adolescent period. These include transitions from junior to more senior schools, and school to work environments. Some of these transitions, particularly that to junior high school, has received considerable research attention, at least in the United States (Simmons & Blyth 1987; Eccles & Midgley 1989). Any transition can be associated with difficulties for some individuals, especially if there is a mis-match between the individual's readiness for the transition and the new environment. Adolescents changing to junior high in the 7th grade (aged 13 years), show greater decrements in self-esteem than those changing in 8th grade. Losses in self-esteem that occur for the younger group do not appear to be recovered significantly during the high-school years. Simmons and Blyth (1987) suggest a *developmental readiness hypothesis*, such that children can be forced into new environments before they are sufficiently mature to handle the implicit social demands.

The school transition poses most problems for early maturing girls (Simmons & Blyth 1987). They are most dissatisfied with their body-image, have lower levels of self-esteem, and seem least able to deal with the social expectations and greater independence demanded from them. Consequently, Simmons and Blyth (1987) stress the inter-dependence between pubertal development and ability to make successful transitions within the school context.

Implications for adolescents' health care

First, there may be some disadvantage for adolescents in basing decisions about the *timing* of the transition on physiological maturity. Certainly in the context of school-based transitions, early maturing girls seem to be at some disadvantage. This may be attributable to the fact that early maturing girls may be less prepared psychologically to deal with the increased demands for independence and responsibility that are associated with adult-based clinics. Their physical maturity may deceive themselves and their physicians into false expectations about their readiness for as complete independence as is generally demanded. Decisions about the timing of transitions need to be made as much on estimates of adolescents' psychological as on their physical maturity. Factors which contribute to psychological readiness to transfer, as suggested by Cappelli *et al.* (1989) need to be identified and refined.

Second, there are indications that adolescent girls experience more difficulties in transferring clinics (Salmi *et al.* 1986) and perceive diabetes to impose greater restrictions on their lives generally (Challen *et al.* 1988) compared with boys. Females tend to know more about diabetes compared with males, and this greater knowledge may contribute to more insight into the possible consequences of the disease and heightened anxiety. In addition, it may be that females find it more difficult to fit their own treatment demands around other peoples' schedules. This can become particularly difficult for a young mother with diabetes who finds that the demands of a young baby for food and care take precedence over her own self-care needs. Future work needs to be directed toward unraveling the processes whereby diabetes differentially affects males and females.

Third, it is apparent that for many patients, the transition from pediatric to adult care almost corresponds to a 'rite of passage', and as such can be viewed as part of a natural and highly desirable shift to adulthood, paralleling the shift from school to work, or leaving the parental home for independent living. For a small number of patients, however, the transition is more fraught. It is apparent that some patients use the opportunity to opt out of care altogether, (at least temporarily). It is particularly for these patients that care needs to be taken to ease the practical arrangements for transition, and that obvious differences between clinics are minimized. Pediatricians and adult physicians need to be aware of potential differences in approach which may jeopardize patients' preparedness to accept hospital based care.

Adolescence is a time of many transitions; physiological, hormonal, psychological and environmental. In considering the type of service that is provided for adolescents, attention needs to be paid to all of these factors, as well as the interplay between them.

CHAPTER 5
Concepts of Stress and Coping

In previous chapters, the impact of chronic disease has been described in relation to children's developmental status. Children's concerns, behaviour and attitudes toward the disease must be considered within a theoretical framework which takes into account the known cognitive, social and emotional changes associated with normal development. Very young children will take their lead from their parents' example; parents who have always been anxious about hospitals are likely to communicate this to their children. As they grow up, other people assume greater importance in influencing children, especially teachers and peers. Older still, it is not so much that children take their cues from parents, as that they become adept at hiding their feelings. Parents, and children in their turn attempt to protect each other from awareness of each other's feelings. Added to their concerns about the illness is an awareness among some children that they can use aspects of the disease to control the behaviour of others; teachers, parents and peers. This can be used to protect others, as in the case of children with life- threatening conditions who pretend to be ignorant of the implications of the disease, or confrontational, where children realise that they have considerable power by refusing medication or faking seizures.

Children's concerns about illness become more social as they grow up (Millstein, Adler & Irwin 1981). Small children may like the idea of staying home and playing with toys; older children worry that they will fall behind in school-work or miss social functions. Small children worry about being separated from parents; older children about whether treatment will hurt, or that their friends will forget about them.

While concerns about illness change throughout childhood, the ability to cope with these concerns and the practical consequences of disease (for example, not crying during treatment, or managing to fit lengthy treatments around homework and social activities) also changes. This chapter is specifically about developmental changes in children's perceptions of stressors associated with disease and their resources for coping. Recent theoretical models emphasise the importance of coping resources and strategies in promoting good adjustment to chronic disease. In this chapter, I will attempt to describe and assess more systematically these models of 'coping'.

Theoretical models of coping

'Coping' has proved an illusory concept to define and quantify, but most current opinion adopts some aspects of that proposed by Lazarus and Folkman (1984):

> 'Constantly changing cognitive and behavioural efforts to manage specific external and/or internal demands that are appraised as taxing or exceeding the resources of the person' (p.144).

Compas, Worsham and Ey (1992) identified four approaches to studying coping in children and adolescence. These include the *Cognitive-appraisal* model (Lazarus & Folkman 1984); the *Primary-secondary control* model (Rothbaum, Weisz & Snyder 1982); the *Ego-psychological* model (Murphy & Moriarty 1976) and the *Monitoring-blunting* model (Miller 1980). All four models make the assumption that coping can be construed in two ways. Individuals can attempt to cope 1) by attempting to change or control some aspect of the individual or environment or 2) by managing or regulating the negative emotions associated with the stressor. The first type of coping is described as 'problem-focussed' by Lazarus and Folkman; as 'primary-control' by Rothbaum, Weisz and Snyder; as 'approach-coping' by Murphy and Moriarty and as 'monitoring' by Miller. The second type of coping has been described in the respective models as 'emotion-focussed'; 'secondary-control'; 'avoidance' and 'blunting'.

As an example, consider a child with cystic fibrosis who is told that it is necessary to undergo physiotherapy on a daily basis. The child may cope by controlling the time when this happens or by becoming very knowledgeable about the disease. This would be considered a form of problem-focussed coping, in that the child is making efforts to master as many aspects of care and treatment as possible. Another child might respond by attempting to deal with the negative emotions aroused by the need for physiotherapy. This might include efforts to relax or play down the importance of the treatment. A child with diabetes, adopting a problem-focussed approach to managing the diet, might become very knowledgeable about the value of different foods. In order to cope with injections, the child adopting an emotion-focussed approach may decide to relax before injecting insulin.

Sub-types of coping

This broad based distinction between problem- and emotion-focussed coping has proved in practice to need some refinement. A number of taxonomies have been developed, especially in work with adults

(Carver, Scheier & Weintraub 1989). These authors distinguished 13 different conceptual strategies. Subtypes of problem-focussed coping included *active coping,* increasing one's efforts and trying to cope in a step wise fashion; *planning,* thinking and coming up with action strategies; *suppression of competing strategies,* not being distracted and putting aside other tasks, and *restraint coping,* not acting prematurely. *Seeking social support* is an additional form of problem focussed coping, especially where the support is sought for specific, practical purposes.

Individuals can also *seek social support for emotional purposes,* by looking for moral support, sympathy or understanding. Individuals can sometimes be reassured by the social support of others. But this strategy can also be maladaptive, to the extent that individuals can use social support as a means of venting their anger. Focussing and venting of emotions can be maladaptive especially where the individual comes to brood on problems. *Behavioural and emotional disengagement* can also be maladaptive, by impeding active coping efforts. A further type of emotion focussed coping includes *positive reinterpretation and growth. Denial* is often thought to be useful in the early stages of stress, but becomes less adaptive later. The opposite is *acceptance,* frequently seen to be a coming to terms with the stressor and realistic attempts to live with the situation. Finally, many people *turn to religion,* which may be a form of emotion focussed coping, in that it allows the individual to reappraise the situation and develop psychologically. It can also be more problem focussed, in that the members of the church may be available for practical as well as emotional support.

While the gross distinction between problem- and emotion- focussed coping is also inadequate when considering the efforts made by children and adolescents, developmental differences preclude the adoption of distinctions such as these made with respect to adult coping (Compas 1987). Work with children has been handicapped because distinctions within the broad based problem/emotion focussed coping have only recently been acknowledged. There has also been a tendency to concentrate on children's theoretical responses to questions about their coping strategies, that is a focus on what they think they might do in any situation, rather than what they actually would do in any specific instance.

Developmental patterns in children's use of coping strategies
Developmental changes have been reported in children's use of different coping strategies across a range of everyday stressors. The normal methodology employed in these studies involves asking children to identify the best way of coping with one of two types of imagined stressor. Some researchers present children with a short list of potential

stressors (having to take an exam, read a passage aloud to the class, visit the dentist, have a routine injection). Others also ask children to identify a situation which was stressful to them. Children might want to include recent arguments with parents or siblings, or failing to get as good a grade as they had hoped in a test. Children are usually asked how frequently these situations create problems for them, and how they would deal with them.

There are no consistent findings with regard to developmental changes in problem-focussed coping. Decreases in use of problem-focussed coping were noted with age in two studies which focussed on strategy-use in relation to medical stressors (going to the doctor or dentist) (Band & Weisz 1988; Curry & Russ 1985). However, where children have been asked about a wider range of stressors, including school – rather than medical situations, no changes in preferences for problem-focussed coping have been reported (Altshuler & Ruble 1989; Compas, Malcarne & Fondacaro 1988). Greater consistency has emerged in relation to the development of emotion-focussed coping, which appears to increase with age, and this applies to both medical (Band & Weisz 1988) and non-medical stressors (Compas, Malcarne & Fondacaro 1988).

In reviewing this literature, Compas, Worsham and Ey (1992) make two important points. The first is that the earlier development of problem-focussed coping can be relatively parsimoniously explained in terms of the ease with which these strategies are modelled by adults in the child's environment and can be observed by the child. Emotion-focussed coping strategies may develop later because they are far less obvious or easy for the child to observe. In addition, children may only slowly become aware that emotions can be brought under personal control. The second point is that, despite its later development, it should not be assumed that emotion-focussed coping is superior to problem-focussed coping. Indeed, it can be associated with many disadvantages. Compas, Malcarne and Fondacaro (1988) reported that children who adopted emotion-focussed styles of coping with non-medical stressors, were also rated as having more emotional and behavioural problems than those who adopted more problem- focussed perspectives.

Coping with medical stressors

A number of studies have attempted to describe the coping strategies used by children with chronic disease to manage painful aspects of the treatment regimen. Band (1990) asked children with diabetes how they attempted to help themselves cope with the pain or frequency of having to deal with dietary restrictions, blood-tests, and insulin injections. The coding criteria adopted followed the theoretical distinctions outlined above, i.e. children's responses were coded as primary or secondary. A third distinction of *relinquished control* or failed coping, was also made. Children were asked about the perceived goal of different coping strategies. So for each coping strategy described, they were asked *how* this made them feel better. Responses were coded as *instrumental* (a specific behaviour), *cognitive*, or *social-emotional* (interpersonal). Younger children were more likely to use primary control than older children. More important, children who relied on primary control appeared to be better adjusted and accepting of the disease and treatment than children who relied on secondary control.

Gil *et al.* (1992) assessed coping strategies in children with sickle cell disease. Children who reported a greater number of different coping strategies were more physically active and required less frequent health care. Those who relied more often on emotion-focussed coping (passive avoidance and catastrophizing) were less active, required more frequent health care interventions and were generally more distressed during procedures.

The assessment of coping in children

A problem to date is the variability in ways in which coping strategies have been categorised, limiting the extent to which comparisons can be made across studies. The development of KIDCOPE may go some way in overcoming this problem. Separate versions of this scale have been developed for younger (aged 7–12 years) and older children (aged 13–18 years). The KIDCOPE assesses the frequency and perceived efficacy of ten commonly used cognitive and behavioural strategies (see table 5.1)

Table 5.1 Examples of responses and categories of coping assessed by KIDCOPE (from Spirito, Stark & Tyc 1989)

Category	Examples of responses
Distraction	I just tried to forget it
Social withdrawal	I stayed by myself
Cognitive restructuring	I tried to see the good side of things
Self-criticism	I blamed myself for causing the problem
Blaming others	I blamed someone else
Problem-solving	I tried to do something to fix the problem
Emotion regulation	I tried to calm myself down
Wishful-thinking	I wished I could make things different
Social support	I tried to talk to others
Resignation	I did nothing as nothing can change things

Spirito, Stark and Tyc (1989) included children with a range of chronic diseases in their assessment of the value of the KIDCOPE in identifying coping strategies in this population. Children were first asked to think of a health-related problem that had occurred within the last month, and rate their emotional response to it. They then completed the KIDCOPE with regard to that problem, indicating how often and how useful the different strategies were in dealing with the problem. In addition to medical problems, children were asked to think of a non-medical problem and complete the KIDCOPE again.

Females used more coping strategies generally, as well as more emotion focussed coping strategies than males. In a related study, Spirito *et al.* (1988) found that children with chronic disease who were referred for emotional help were more likely to report using distraction, social withdrawal and wishful thinking compared with children with chronic disease but not referred for help. This result appears to imply that reliance on these strategies is non- adaptive and further that interventions should encourage children to adopt more problem, rather than emotion-focussed coping.

Again based on findings using the KIDCOPE, Stark, Spirito and Tyc (1991) argued that the assessment of stress and coping strategies in chronically sick children should go beyond an analysis of strategies used to deal with pain. Among chronically sick children, only 33 per cent described 'pain' as their main problem. Half the total sample selected some other aspect of hospitalization as their main problem (for example, not being able to sleep at night; lack of privacy or poor food), and 17 per cent selected some aspect of their diagnosis (concern about prognosis or course of the disease). Overall, some changes in preference for different coping strategies were noted. Problem-solving and wishful-thinking were used more frequently by older children, anxious or sad children. Chronically ill adolescents used self- blame and wishful thinking less often than younger, chronically ill children.

Coping strategies adopted by parents

Despite the difficulties that face families with a child with chronic disease, many continue to function with the minimum of disruption, and are not distinguishable from other families. In many ways, this is a remarkable achievement. How is it that some families appear devastated by the illness, while others take it in their stride? The clinical literature suggests that families who cope adopt particular strategies. For example, they may cope by turning to God, making positive efforts to look for 'good' things that have come out of the child's disease, such as helping them accept each other for what they are, or being less personally ambitious. Others are assumed to cope by 'denial' – essentially not allowing knowledge of the disease to interfere very much with their everyday lives. It is not clear how wide-spread these methods of coping may be; nor if some strategies are very much more common or successful than others.

There are many myths about coping. It is often assumed that any kind of loss or illness is initially responded to by grief and mourning, and that recovery occurs slowly over a period of time. In response to the diagnosis of chronic childhood disease, or death of a child, it has been assumed that individuals go through a series of 'stages' (Horowitz & Kaltreider 1980; Kübler-Ross 1969). These stage-based models often lead to expectations that there are 'right' and 'wrong' ways of responding to crises, and any deviation from these defined paths are indicative of psychopathology. Based on extensive work with adults who experience a wide range of trauma, Wortman and Silver (1987) have shown that many individuals continue to experience distress over long periods of time, and these distresses can be exacerbated by special occasions like birthdays or anniversaries, as well as being aggravated by unexpected events or memories. Coping with chronic disease is not a linear process, but instead families face a series of 'ups' and 'downs' (Spinetta 1981).

In relation to chronic childhood disease, one of the most systematic attempts to describe, measure and assess the implications of different coping strategies has been made by McCubbin et al. (1983). These authors developed the Coping Health Inventory for Parents (CHIP) specifically to measure coping strategies adopted by families with a child with chronic disease. The original scale consisted of 45 items, chosen to assess general response to stress. In addition, other items were drawn from;

- *Network and Social support theory* (reflecting the family's relationship to the community and each other for emotional and social support);

- *Family Stress theory* (management of intra- and inter-family dynamics in adjusting to treatment management and normal growth and development of the child);

- *Individual coping* (psychological adjustment needed to manage anxiety and emotion);

- *Family medical support* (parents' efforts to communicate with medical staff and other parents, and master practical aspects of medical care).

Three positive coping patterns were identified from parents' responses on the CHIP. The first, *maintaining family integration, cooperation and an optimistic definition* of the situation, was made up of 19 items reflecting behaviours that focus on the family's beliefs about life and the disease, encourage cooperation and involvement between family members, and foster independence. The second pattern, *maintaining social support, self-esteem and psychological stability*, consisted of 18 items reflecting parents' efforts to obtain a sense of well-being through the social support of others. The third coping pattern, *understanding the medical situation through communication with other parents and medical staff*, consisted of 8 items relating to interactions and communication between parents and medical staff.

Nevin, McCubbin and Birkebak (1983) found that mothers of children with cerebral palsy or myelomingocele emphasised the role of the family, the relationship between family and medical staff, and the opportunity to talk to friends as specially helpful in coping with the child's condition. Fathers, in contrast, emphasised the importance of family stability, keeping themselves in good shape, and doing things together with their spouse and children.

Differences in coping between mothers and fathers when a newborn needs intensive care

As described in Chapter 2, having a baby in intensive care is a very stressful event for parents, yet there appears to be consistent differences between mothers and fathers in the way in which these stresses are handled.

Affleck *et al.* (1990) compared 50 mothers and their partners with infants in an intensive care unit in terms of coping strategies and emotional responses. In addition to describing coping strategies adopted separately by mothers and fathers, they also attempted to consider the relation between coping strategies adopted by one partner for the mental health of the other.

Mothers of infants requiring intensive care were more emotionally disturbed than fathers, although a number of variables appeared to influence these differences in reported stress levels. Mothers anticipated more health problems for their child in the future compared with fathers. Mothers appeared less able to adopt effective coping strategies and fathers appeared adept at minimizing the depth of their feelings. In addition, too, many mothers may have been experiencing post-partum depression or recovering from surgery themselves, which may have heightened their emotional concern generally.

Mothers and fathers shared some views about the impact of the experience of intensive care. Both agreed about the harm that was associated with the stay in intensive care, (i.e. parents gave similar ratings to statements such as 'My relationship with my child has been harmed by this experience', 'This experience is one of the worst things that could happen to anyone'). Parents agreed less about the potential benefits of the experience, i.e they did not agree on statements such as 'My life has taken a turn for the better since this happened', 'My baby is more precious to me because of what we went through together'.

Despite mothers' higher levels of emotional distress, they were not as effective as fathers in mobilizing effective coping strategies. Mothers were more likely to adopt social support or escapist coping strategies, (turning to others for emotional support and indulging in wishful thinking or day-dreaming). Fathers adopted more effective strategies whereby they were able to minimize the perceived threat of the situation, or take some concerted action to improve things. The success of these strategies is reflected in more positive mood experiences of fathers.

Most mothers and fathers acknowledged differences between them in the way in which they attempted to cope with the crisis. However, there were differences in their evaluations of each others attempts to cope, with many couples acknowledging the potential benefits of complementary coping strategies.

As is discussed further in Chapter 6, fathers of chronically sick children are invariably assigned a supportive role; that is, they are encouraged to respond by helping the mother to cope rather than assume primary responsibility themselves. Affleck, Tennen and Rowe (1990) acknowledged that this was the way in which many couples attempted to deal with the crisis, but stress the potential benefits of mutual supportive processes.

While research using CHIP has generally been concerned with the implications of parents' coping strategies for their own health or behaviour, a study by Sanger, Copeland and Davidson (1991) suggests that different strategies may have implications for the way in which children themselves function. In a sample of 48 children with cancers, the frequency of somatic complaints and academic difficulties were both high. However, within the group, difficulties were associated with gender, social competence and parent coping. Boys experienced more difficulties than girls. Children with most difficulties came from families in which parents reported fewer coping strategies. Parents who tried to maintain family organisation, cooperated and remained optimistic about the disease had children who were rated as better adjusted (by a parent). The authors concluded that parents who remain hopeful are able, through modelling, to promote positive coping strategies in their children, though it would of course be necessary to obtain independent ratings of children's adjustment in future studies. (Parents who rate their own coping as good or successful may be more likely to rate their children as well adjusted compared with parents who feel they are not coping so well).

The relationship between preferred coping strategy and disease

Given the diverse practical and emotional demands associated with different chronic diseases, there is every reason to suppose that parents may find some strategies more helpful when dealing with some diseases compared with others. For example, given the demands of self-care, the need to understand the rationale for treatment and develop practical skills in implementing treatment is much greater when a child has diabetes or cystic fibrosis compared with other conditions. It might therefore be expected that parents would be more likely to report that finding out about the disease and seeking information would be helpful. In contrast, it may be far less helpful to learn more about cancer, since there is little that parents can do in the way of nursing care for their child, and it is more likely that information would centre on the life-threatening nature of the disease. Parents of children with cancer may therefore find it not helpful to learn a great deal about the disease.

Eiser and Havermans (1992) used an Anglicised version of CHIP to compare coping strategies reported to be helpful by parents of children suffering from one of five conditions (diabetes, asthma, cardiac disease, epilepsy and leukemia). The scales were completed independently by mothers and fathers. In addition, parents were asked to rate the degree to which the disease was associated with difficulties in fifteen different aspects of their lives. These included practical difficulties related to where the family lived or how they chose furnishings for their home, and more personal difficulties, such as limiting time for sports and hobbies or opportunities to be with other children and friends. The study was therefore concerned to identify any differences between mothers and fathers in the coping strategies they found most helpful, and to describe ways in which strategies were dependent on the degree of difficulties parents perceived to be associated with the disease.

A principal components factor analysis of the coping scale resulted in a four factor solution, which was essentially the same for mothers' and fathers' ratings considered separately. Factor 1 appeared to be best described in terms of *autonomy*, and included items such as 'involve myself in social activities', 'get away by myself', and 'keep myself well-groomed and in shape'. Factor 2 was labelled a *medical care* factor, since it included items such as 'believe my child is getting the best medical care possible' and 'believe my child will get better'. Factor 3 was labelled *social support and information* and included items such as 'read more about the medical condition' and 'talk to other parents in the same situation and learn from their experiences'. The fourth factor, *family-support*, included items such as 'do things together as a family' and 'get other members of the family to help with chores and tasks at home'.

As we hypothesised, parents' reports of the extent to which the different coping strategies were helpful was dependent on the particular disease. Parents of children with epilepsy and cardiac conditions found *autonomy* to be more helpful than parents in the other groups, while parents of children with leukemia reported this to be the least helpful. *Medical care* was rated as most helpful by parents of children with cardiac conditions, while parents of children with diabetes and epilepsy reported that *social support* was a more helpful strategy than parents in the other conditions. Parents of children with epilepsy and leukemia were least likely to find *family-support* a helpful strategy.

There were no real differences in the helpfulness of different coping strategies as a function of time since diagnosis. However, there were some differences between mothers and fathers. Mothers tended to endorse all items more than fathers, with the biggest differences being on the *social support* and *medical care* factors.

With regard to disease related difficulties, mothers reported more difficulties than fathers. Neither the child's age nor time since diagnosis, were related to the degree of difficulties reported. Mothers of girls perceived themselves to experience fewer difficulties than mothers of boys. Mothers and fathers of children with leukemia reported more difficulties than parents in any other group. Least difficulties were reported by parents of children with diabetes and cardiac conditions. Intermediate levels were reported by parents of those with epilepsy and asthma.

Finally, Eiser and Havermans (1992) considered whether parents' perceptions of disease related difficulties influenced their endorsement of the different coping strategies. For mothers, greater perceived difficulties were associated with stronger endorsement of the *social support* factor, i.e. the more mothers felt there were difficulties associated with the disease the more they reported that they relied on social support. For these women, the more difficulties they experienced caring for the sick child the more they found it helpful to talk to others in a similar position. For fathers, more perceived difficulties were associated with stronger endorsement of the *autonomy* factor, that is, the more difficulties fathers experienced, the more they felt it important to keep themselves fit or throw themselves into their work. There was also a marginal, inverse relationship with the *medical care* factor. This applied to both mothers and fathers, but was stronger for fathers, and suggests that the more difficulties the family experience, the less they perceive interactions or support from medical staff to be *helpful*.

There are some problems in interpreting these data, since it is not clear exactly how parents interpreted the meaning of the instructions 'to rate the items in terms of how helpful you find these different ways of coping'. Consider the item 'talk with the doctor about my concerns about my child'. Parents might rate this as 'not very helpful' because whenever they ask questions they have difficulty understanding what is said, or prefer not to think about some of the issues raised. Alternatively, parents might rate the item as 'not helpful' because, even though they would actually find it helpful to talk to the doctor, the opportunity does not actually arise. So they may perceive the strategy to be helpful in the abstract, but in practice feel that they have little, or insufficient experience with it. This problem raises the question as to whether fathers who perceive there to be more difficulties associated with the child's condition really perceive medical support to be less helpful, or if they are more realistic than mothers in accepting that little can be done to really the change the situation.

Appraisal of disease related stress

As was described in the introduction, caring for a child with chronic disease is associated with a substantial increase in the number of stressful situations with which parents have to deal. Successful management of the disease requires that families learn new strategies in order to reduce the practical stresses involved to manageable proportions. Much of the early literature was concerned with describing disease related stresses, and it was generally concluded that families lacked the resources to deal effectively with many of the stresses imposed on them.

This deficit-centered approach has been very much challenged more recently (Drotar & Crawford 1985). One reason for this is theoretical. The early focus on psychoanalytic theory has generally been superseded by more cognitive orientations. This theoretical change has been associated with a shift from interest in what can go wrong in an individual's efforts to cope, to one in which there is greater interest in how individuals construe their environment and make active efforts to restore a degree of equilibrium. Workers such as Rutter (1981), Garmezy *et al.* 1984 and others have done much to bring concepts of 'resilience' to the forefront of our understanding. At the same time, participants in research are not exclusively those who have already been referred to clinical agencies for some pathological reason. Rather, efforts are made to involve a cross-section of a total clinic population, so that the study group includes a representative sample of families.

Second, there has been a shift in the type of methodologies employed, and particularly a move away from clinic type interviews to the more routine use of standardized questionnaires. This has meant that there has been some effort to elicit positive or more adaptive strategies of coping, rather than make the more simplistic assumption that chronic disease is inevitably associated with malfunction.

Third, a number of studies have challenged the earlier position that families of children with chronic disease are more likely to exhibit psychopathology compared with families of healthy children. Some reports suggested that mothers of chronically ill children were no more depressed than mothers of healthy children (Kronenberger & Thompson 1990); siblings of chronically sick children were not substantially different from siblings of healthy children (Drotar & Crawford 1985), and in several reviews, it was concluded that the children themselves showed few measurable deficits as measured by examination successes (Malpas 1988) or more social aspects of functioning. Further-more, it was suggested that it was possible to identify *positive* effects of chronic disease. Some families reported that their lives had improved, in that they were now more considerate of each other and felt closer together (Johnson 1980). Siblings, too, seemed to derive something good from the situation; often showing greater empathy and consideration towards others in more mature and sympathetic ways than children who did not have a chronically sick sibling (Horwitz & Kazak 1990).

In order to account for these divergent findings, it has been suggested that families differ in the way in which they *perceive* the stresses associated with the disease (Lazarus & Folkman 1984; Wallander *et al.* 1989). Some families may feel that it is not so much trouble to do the extra cleaning necessary where a child with asthma is allergic to dust, while others may find this to be a real strain; either because they hate housework, or because they live in poor accommodation which is almost impossible to keep clean anyway. Some mothers may take in their stride the fact that their child needs more care than others of the same age, while other mothers resent these continual demands.

In an attempt to quantify the stresses experienced by parents of chronically sick children, Abidin and Burke (1978) outlined a schematic representation of the variables which might potentially contribute to the appraisal of stress (see table 5.2). This schema became the basis for the development of the Parenting Stress Index (PSI), (Abidin 1983). This is a self-report scale, designed specifically to assess parental stress in relation to child-rearing. Three major domains of stress can be derived; relating to child characteristics, parent characteristics and general life-stress. In the *child* domain, adaptability, acceptability, demandingness, mood, distractibility, and reinforcement of the parent are the key concepts assessed. Examples of items included to measure these dimensions include:

'My child gets upset easily over the smallest thing' (adaptability);

'My child does a few things which bother me a great deal' (acceptability);

'Most times I feel my child likes me and wants to be close to me' (reinforcement of parents).

In the *parent* domain, depression, attachment to the child, role-restriction, sense of competence, social isolation, relationship between the spouses and parent health are assessed. Example items include:

'I feel trapped by my responsibilities as a parent' (role restrictions);

'Since having my child, my spouse has not given me as much support as I expected' (relationships with spouse);

'I feel that I am a good parent' (sense of competence).

General life stress included 19 items, none of which were related to the child's health; (moving house; separations, etc.) The scale shows good internal reliability and consistency over a one year period (Abidin 1983), and has been used in a considerable amount of research concerned with parenting stresses. Some limitations of the scale have recently been acknowledged (Abidin 1990). These largely stem from assumptions prevalent in the early 1980s about the nature of stress. Parent distress was then conceptualized as a continuous linear outcome variable for which chronic disease was considered the most significant cause. Parents of chronically sick children were seen to experience multiple stresses which eventually exceeded their abilities to cope. At this threshold, parents experienced significant levels of stress. More recent work points to the variability and inconsistencies in experienced stress, suggesting that a complex system of disease and situational factors are determinants of experienced stress.

'Caretaking burden is multidimensional and encompasses variables ranging from the dependency of the ill child to the availability of alternative caretakers' (Hauenstein 1990, p.361).

Early models failed to acknowledge individual differences in parents' personality, cognitions, or perceptions which mediated perceived and experienced stress. Although this scale has been used extensively, it is very negative in orientation, giving parents little opportunity to describe any positive experiences.

Disease-specific stressors

A number of studies found no differences between parents of sick and healthy children in terms of the levels of stress reported either on the

Table 5.2 Model of theoretical pathways linking parenting behaviour and child outcomes (from Abidin & Burke 1978)

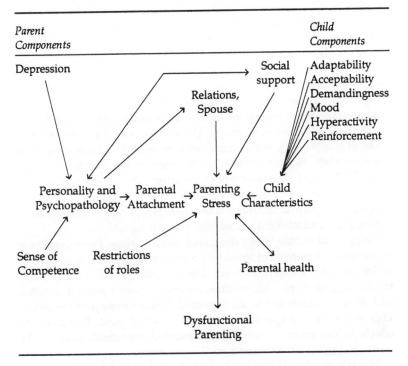

Parenting Stress Index (Bendell *et al.* 1986; Kazak & Marvin 1984; Kazak, Reber & Snitzer 1988; Hauenstein *et al.* 1989) or on any other measure of stress outcome (Walker, Ford & Donald 1987). However, in most of these studies, parents of ill children scored higher than parents of healthy children on scales measuring general stress. Mothers of sick children tended to have lower scores than comparison mothers on scales assessing child characteristics and parental self-esteem and competence. Thus, although 'not significant', careful study of these data suggest, as would be expected, that parents of chronically sick children experienced more day-to-day stresses than parents of healthy children. (Such a conclusion is substantiated by research suggesting elevated levels of anxiety and depression in mothers of chronically sick children; see Chapter 6 for review).

Other studies have reported elevated stress levels in families of chronically sick children (Goldberg *et al.* (1990). Two groups of chronically sick children were included; 15 families with an infant with cystic fibrosis and 26 with an infant with congenital heart disease. Both groups were compared with a group of healthy infants and their parents. On assessment, all infants were under one year of age. The three groups of parents did not differ in their ratings of general life stress. However, there were significant differences on five of the six child domains described above. Parents of healthy children reported least stress in relation to their child ratings, and parents of those with congenital heart disease the most. Parents of infants with cystic fibrosis were most likely to report that stress was increased due to the child's demandingness.

In terms of the parent domains, two dimensions differentiated most clearly between the three groups. These were parent depression and sense of competence, with parents of normal children reporting least stress on both. Fathers reported more stress in the domains of child distractibility and reinforcement of the parent than mothers. On most parent domains, mothers reported more stress than fathers. The exception was in terms of attachment, where fathers reported more difficulties in forming an attachment to their child than mothers.

Phipps and Drotar (1990) compared ratings on the Parenting Stress Index made by parents of infants on home apnoea monitoring, parents of infants with congenital heart disease, and normal infants. Their results suggested that chronic illness seems to create special difficulties which can be attributed to the increased demandingness of the infant. This in turn may jeopardize parent–infant attachment. However, the effects of the infant's illness and associated demandingness can be off-set by family resources and available supports.

Hauenstein et al. (1989) again used the PSI to study stress levels in parents of children with diabetes. The data for a sub-set of the group were compared against normative data for an age-matched control group. Children with diabetes were perceived to be more demanding than healthy children. In addition, mothers of those with diabetes reported less attachment to their children, less support from their spouse, and poorer health than mothers of healthy children. Yet within the group with diabetes, there was no relationship between reported levels of stress in any of the three domains and the child's metabolic control. Thus, although chronic illness may be associated with increased stress for families, this does not necessarily have adverse implications for the child's physical health.

Levels of stress reported in these and other studies are generally lower than might be expected intuitively, or based on experience with clinical populations. Parents of children with chronic disease tended to report a greater number of stresses, and experienced more ill-health themselves compared with other parents, but the differences between the two groups were not statistically significant. Hauenstein (1990) discusses several reasons to account for the apparent discrepancy between levels of stress which might be expected among families of sick children compared with the levels measured on dimensions of the PSI or related instruments. First, within the PSI, there is an inadequate description of those factors comprising risk and the experience of distress. Processes of parental decision-making, the relationship between decision-making and characteristics of the disease, and consequences for experienced distress, may be more profitably studied. Second, most work focuses on mothers' reports of stress, and it is often unclear if she speaks for herself, or the marital dyad. Certainly, it is not clear how mothers' perceptions of stress relate to fathers' perceptions. Thus, the influence of fathers in decision-making, or their contribution to mothers' perceived stress, is rarely considered. Third, research has seldom considered the implications of parents' stress for the child, parenting efficacy, marital quality, or family stability more generally. Ultimately, the quality of child care is dependent on parents' confidence and ability to implement treatment schedules, and for this reason greater attention should be paid to the consequences of parents' perceived stress. This points to the potentially greater value of using the PSI to describe differences in perceived stress levels within populations having the same disease, rather than compare across disease groups, or with 'normal' controls. Measures such as the PSI should be useful in relating levels of experienced stress to outcome variables, and thus may go towards accounting for the differential responses characteristic of families coping with apparently the same conditions.

Some evidence of the relationship between perceived stress and emotional outcome for the child is reported by DeMaso *et al.* (1991). Mothers of 99 children with congenital heart disease completed measures of child adjustment, the PSI, and also rated their beliefs about the severity of the child's condition. Mothers of well-adjusted children were themselves less depressed and reported more emotional closeness and empathy with their child. These mothers described themselves as competent and were not resentful towards their children. Within the child domain, greater stress levels were reported by single parents or those with younger children, regardless of perceived or objective disease severity. However, children with more severe disease were perceived to be less reinforcing to parents.

Distinctions also need to be made between stresses that affect all parents, and those that apply specifically to those caring for a child with chronic disease. Quittner (1992) compared parents' reports of stresses depending on whether the child had a hearing impairment or a seizure disorder, in relation to those with a healthy child. Mothers of hearing impaired children and those with a seizure disorder rated their children as more demanding, moody and distractible than mothers rated their healthy children. They also reported more behaviour problems, and experienced greater difficulties with family routines and activities. Mothers of hearing impaired children reported more stress, over and above mothers of those with a seizure disorder. Qualitative differences occurred in the nature of stressors reported by mothers depending on the child's condition.

Mothers of deaf children reported greater stresses in relation to language training, communication and finding an appropriate educational placement. Mothers of those with a seizure disorder were more concerned about safety, medication and controlling seizures. Mothers of healthy children rated most important stresses as sibling rivalry, toilet training, mealtimes and bedtimes.

Perceptions of severity

According to Lazarus and Folkman (1984) the individual's appraisal of the stress of a situation rather than the 'objective' measure of stress is important in determining response. This hypothesis suggests that mothers' beliefs about the severity of the child's condition will be more influential and predictive of her behaviour than medical indices of severity. Certainly, there is little evidence that objective indices of medical severity are predictive of mothers' behaviour or child adjustment, (Carr, Pearson & Halliwell 1983; Lavigne, Nolan & McLone 1988; Wallander et al. 1989).

There is, however, some evidence that mothers' perceptions of the severity of the child's condition is a powerful predictor of her own, the family and the child's adjustment. Perhaps the classic example of the influence of individual perceptions of disease severity on behaviour was reported by Linde and colleagues (Linde, Rosof & Dunn 1970; Linde et al. 1966) in mothers of children with congenital heart disease. Children who were misdiagnosed as infants were subsequently found to be protected and restricted in their activities in much the same way as children who were correctly identified with heart murmers. Thus, parents' behaviour was determined by their beliefs about the child's condition, rather than any physical limitations in the child.

More recently, DeMaso et al. (1991) reported that mothers' perceptions of the severity of the child's heart condition was an important predictor of the child's adjustment. Mothers' perceptions of severity were based on measures of locus of control, and stress and ratings of severity (from insignificant to severe). Indices of medical severity were derived from medical records, and included number and frequency of admissions, number of operations and cardiac catheterizations and on-going problems (rated by a nurse clinician). Specific heart lesions were recorded, and the Cardiologists' Perception of Medical Severity used to assess medical severity. These indices of perceived and medical severity were used to predict childrens' adjustment. Approximately 33 per cent of the variability in adjustment was accounted for by mothers' ratings of severity, with only 3 per cent being accounted for by ratings of severity derived from medical indices. Thus, the severity of the heart lesion itself bore no relationship to mothers' beliefs about the child's behaviour and adjustment.

In other studies, too, there is evidence for the relatively greater importance of perceived severity over more objective indices. In epilepsy, for example, the degree to which individual family members perceived there to be disruption following a seizure was more predictive of family adjustment than the actual amount of disruption that occurred (Appolone-Ford, Gibson & Driefuss 1983).

Eiser *et al.* (1991b) compared mothers' and fathers' ratings of the severity of asthma in their pre-school children in relation to more objective estimates based on prescribed drugs and their frequency of administration. A 'mildly' affected group (n=19) received treatment medication only 'as necessary'. A 'moderately' affected group (n=18) received daily prophylactic medication. Six children in this group were regularly treated by courses of oral steroids. The groups also differed in number of hospitalizations and length of admission; both of these being greater in the 'moderate' group. Mothers and fathers were separately asked to rate their own perception of the severity of the child's asthma, and indicate the extent to which they believed asthma attacks were caused by common precipitating factors (such as dust, exercise, food, animals, colds or emotion).

Ratings of perceived severity made by mothers and fathers correlated with severity assessed by medication. However, there was no significant correlation between mothers' and fathers' ratings of perceived severity, nor any agreement between them about factors which precipitated asthma attacks in their child. Fathers perceived their children to be more severely affected than mothers. There were some associations between parents' ratings of severity and their perceptions of, and behaviour towards, the sick child. Mothers reported that mildly affected children were less affectionate, and more difficult to deal with especially when out shopping or visiting. Fathers of the mildly affected group rated their children as less likely to do as they were told or to enjoy life than fathers of the moderately affected.

However, there is no simple relationship between mothers' perceptions of severity and behavioural factors (at least in asthma). Perrin, MacLean and Perrin (1989) found that the adjustment of children with asthma was rated as worse by parents who rated the severity of the disease as 'moderate'. Children described by their parents as 'mildly' or 'severely' affected were rated as better adjusted. Parents' perceptions of adjustment therefore, may be affected by expectations about appropriate behaviour. Adjustment may be rated as better when the child is very ill because parents' expectations are very low. In contrast, where children are mildly affected, parents may have high expectations which are rarely achieved.

Coping or surviving?

The current emphasis on coping is welcome, and an improvement over very traditional approaches which stressed the maladjustment and difficulties experienced by families in bringing up a child with chronic disease. Perhaps there is a danger that we are moving too far in this direction. The fact that some families clearly manage very well can lead us to expect that this should be the norm, and make us less able to empathise with those who find coping more difficult. The sheer numbers of families seen in pediatric clinics also acts to immunize staff against too much involvement. Our culture, too, places considerable value on stoicism and less on any expression of emotional feeling.

Current cognitive approaches to coping is therefore perhaps more idealistic than descriptive of what happens in practice. Although parents can complete measures of coping, like the CHIP, more detailed interviewing often suggests that the helpfulness of different strategies is relative. One kind of strategy may be more helpful than another, but in practice nothing helped very much. Separate interviews with mothers and fathers of children with cancer lead us to this view (Eiser, Havermans & Eiser, 1995). Very few identified specific sources of support, and the support that was available tended to be restricted to specific crisis periods.

'My sister was very helpful at first, but she's got her own life to lead and her own children. We don't see her much now' (Father of child with cancer)

Often people are unable to describe who supported them or how they survived crisis times. One mother felt that God (though I think she meant individuals in the local church) helped her through, but the most frequent response was the need to keep going for the sake of the child and other children in the family. Many parents described themselves as surviving rather than coping. Once treatment is started, the family is on a tread-mill. There is no end, and no possibility of getting off. There may occasionally be decision points, when it is possible not to begin a new course of treatment, but if this opportunity is lost, it is hard to take a decision at any time that treatment is not working. Families cope by virtue of being swept along by the medical system, and few feel they have any control over the direction their lives are taking. There are no choices to be made.

There are separate considerations to be made when discussing strategies children and families can adopt to help them deal with specific practical crises. Some achievements have been made in terms of understanding how children cope with difficulties such as losing their hair, giving themselves daily injections, or eating prescribed foods at determined times. Identifying different strategies in relation to issues such as these is potentially useful, and should form the basis of intervention programs. More esoteric issues, concerned with how children rationalize their situation to themselves, or understand the potentially life-threatening nature of their condition, is less amenable to such cognitive approaches.

This chapter has focussed on coping by children, with some emphasis on parental coping, especially where this has significance for the children themselves. In the following sections, parents' coping and understanding of the disease is considered more specifically, as well as the implications for mothers and fathers separately, and their relationship with each other.

CHAPTER 6

Mothers and Fathers

Mothers' responses to chronic disease in their child

Mothers' responses to chronic disease in their child have received an enormous amount of attention compared with responses of fathers, siblings, and certainly more than members outside the nuclear family, such as grandparents. In part, this bias is for very practical reasons. Mothers traditionally are more involved with child-care, less likely to be employed outside the home, and therefore more frequently able to bring the child to clinic appointments. Concern with mothers' mental health is unfortunately often one of convenience; they tend to be available to take part in research studies during regular working hours.

This view may be unnecessarily cynical, however, since it may also be that mothers are more interested to take part in research, and more likely to see it to be of some potential benefit than fathers. Women place more emphasis on the importance of good family health and see this to be more their responsibility than that of men (Hibbard & Pope 1983). However, as women take on more commitments outside the home and men are encouraged to assume some domestic responsibility, it is important that this is reflected in research. There is a need to involve fathers, in order that we can better understand the processes by which mothers and fathers develop ways of managing and sharing the practical and emotional demands of caring for a child with chronic disease.

Research also needs to move beyond mere descriptions of behaviour. It is not enough to catalogue parents' responses to their child's illness, but essential to consider more carefully the implications of these responses for parent management and understanding of the condition, and, just as importantly, the consequences for the child. Specifically, to what extent are parent and child responses interdependent? There is generally an assumption of consistency in parent and child response, (i.e. that parents who cope well have children who cope well and *vice-versa*), but there is little definitive support for such an hypothesis. Current literature is severely limited in the preoccupation with describing mothers' (and to a far less extent, fathers') attitudes to the illness, and focussing on their differential responsibility for practical aspects of the treatment regimen.

Responsibility for treatment regimens

Caring for any young child takes an inordinate amount of time, much more than most parents expect or are prepared for. The demands escalate where the child has a chronic disease. Following such a diagnosis, parents are obliged to take on many additional responsibilities relating to practical aspects of the treatment regimen. These demands have to be fitted in with other family and work commitments, and can be very time-consuming. There is an assumption (and some evidence) that mothers are more likely to take on responsibility for this extra care than are fathers. It is usually mothers who bring their child for clinic or hospital appointments; rarely fathers (Barbarin, Hughes & Chesler 1988; Drotar, Crawford & Bush 1984; Hobfoll 1991; Willis, Elliott & Jay 1982; DeMaso et al. 1991). In families with a child with diabetes, Zrebiec (1987) showed that much management, including helping the child self-inject insulin or test blood-sugar levels, is the responsibility of mothers rather than fathers. Similarly, Nagy and Ungerer (1990) found that mothers of a child with cystic fibrosis spent longer on childcare and giving physiotherapy than fathers. Cowen et al. (1985) also reported that mothers of children with cystic fibrosis were more responsible for treatment administration than fathers.

Barbarin, Hughes and Chesler (1988) studied 32 families with a child with leukemia. Nineteen (59%) reported that mothers alone were responsible for monitoring the child's care; in 2 families, fathers alone were responsible and in 11 (34%) families both parents shared responsibility. Havermans and Eiser (1991) interviewed mothers of children with spina bifida. All perceived themselves to be much more responsible for the child's care than their husbands, and this applied both to general care-taking as well as more specific tasks associated with the child's disease related restrictions.

Eiser et al. (1991a) found that mothers of pre-school children with asthma were more involved in everyday care compared with fathers. This applied to non-asthma related care, such as washing, feeding or dressing the child. Measures of asthma related care, such as giving medication or taking the child to clinics were not included in this study, but may well further contribute to mothers' burden of care.

In part, the greater responsibility taken by mothers in caring for their sick child may parallel functioning in all families, including those with healthy children (La Rossa 1986). Even where both parents work outside the home, mothers are more responsible for child-rearing tasks than fathers. Where responsibility is measured in terms of *time*, it is generally found that mothers spend more time with their children than fathers.

However, time itself may be inadequate as an indicator of parents' involvement with their children (Greenberger & Goldberg 1989). Where fathers are employed outside the home, it may be very difficult for them to do as much in the way of child- care as they would like. What may be more significant is the extent to which mothers are satisfied with the distribution of labour within the family, or if they feel resentful that the burden of care is shared unequally. (This is discussed again in the section on marital relationships). It is a relatively common complaint that mothers feel alone in caring for the sick child, and that fathers cope by disengaging themselves from family life. Gordon Walker & Manion (1991) found that mothers of children with different chronic conditions reported that they felt much greater responsibility for treatment related care of the child than their husbands, and felt very much alone with this responsibility.

These issues, especially in relation to couples' efforts to care for a terminally ill child, were very much reflected in a report by Cook (1984). Mothers assumed much of the responsibility for daily care. Fathers took a greater responsibility for other siblings and were able to maintain their own self-esteem through their roles as bread-winners. However, Cook (1984) goes on to suggest that these role-differentiations create particular stresses for mothers and fathers. Mothers experienced social isolation and were forced into contact with hospital and medical staff. Fathers reported greater conflict in managing the competing demands of work and the family, and faced increasing isolation from the world of the hospital and dying child. Fathers feared isolation from their child, and were concerned about the toll that care was imposing on their wives.

It is possible that the apparent bias in parents' responsibilities reflects mothers' *perceptions* about the situation, and would not necessarily be endorsed by fathers. It is also possible that parents work out some amicable arrangement between themselves whereby mothers are responsible for the sick child, and fathers for other children in the family. It may be more efficient for mothers to be responsible exclusively for some tasks, and fathers others. By focussing almost exclusively on mothers, and on issues of responsibility in relation to the sick child, it is not clear how parents organize their domestic lives more generally. Only by tackling these issues, however, are we going to gain a more rounded view of how mothers and fathers apportion responsibility for family life generally and care of the sick child more specifically.

How mothers and fathers divide up the care

An interview with the mother of a child with cancer gave the impression that it was she who shouldered all the responsibility for care of the child. It was mum who took the child to clinic, gave medication (which the child resented bitterly), did necessary care and cleaning of the Hickman line, and communicated with the school about the child's absences and health. In fact, this mother described her husband as 'a waste of space'. Yet she was not resentful, and seemed to expect very little of him. His reaction to the child's diagnosis had been one of despair; he was drinking a lot, smoking, and had recently been made redundant because of his 'unreliability'.

Dad was initially reluctant to talk himself, sending a message through his wife that he knew nothing and had other things to do. He took very little persuasion to change his mind. He confirmed that his wife did most of the routine work involved in running the home, looking after other children, and caring for the sick child. At the same time, he saw himself to be very involved with everything that went on in the family, and was very concerned about the child's health. His view about his 'unreliability' was that it was due entirely to his concern about the child, and his frequent visits to the hospital to visit her. He was, in fact, rather derogatory about the way in which his wife cared for the child, feeling that she was too soft, and allowed the child to get away with too many things. His role in the family was therefore very important, in ensuring that treatments were carried out. He never did them himself, but kept his wife on her toes, reminding her, and checking that she carried them out. When the child objected to taking medication, mum apparently would say that there was no harm in waiting, and put off giving medication to avoid an outburst from the child. In contrast, dad's view was that it had to be done, and nothing could be achieved by delay. His role in the family, in his view, was therefore critical; he was ultimately responsible for ensuring that treatments took place.

Mental health and adjustment

Mothers of children with chronic disease are more likely to be anxious and depressed (Breslau, Staruch & Mortimer 1982; Daniels *et al.* 1986; Kronenberger & Thompson 1990), and report more mental and physical health complaints (Wallander *et al.* 1989) compared with mothers of healthy children. This heightened distress should not be surprising. Mothers must deal with the emotional consequences of knowing that the child has a chronic or fatal condition, understand that the child must undergo intense and painful treatments and accept personal responsibility for administering much of this treatment. Mothers sometimes fear that their child will come to hate them for the pain they inflict. At the same time they must deal with the needs of other members of the family, care for other children, and often also attempt to pursue their own careers. Living with this range of stressors is bound to take its toll, and the adverse consequences for mothers' mental and physical health are well documented.

In an early study by McCarthy (1975), for example, one third of a sample of 64 mothers of children with leukemia were being treated with tranquilizers, anti-depressants or sleeping tablets. Insomnia (Lascari & Stehbens 1973; McCarthy 1975), and physical exhaustion (Allan, Townley & Phelan 1974) are also commonly reported.

Although it is clearly established that mothers of chronically sick children commonly show elevated levels of mental health problems, the extent to which this is characteristic of all mothers is less clear. There appear to be particular discrepancies between research based on clinic populations compared with results from larger scale epidemiological surveys. Cadman *et al.* (1991) described the mental health of mothers and fathers of chronically sick and disabled children, drawn from a population of 1869 randomly selected families in Ontario, Canada. Both mothers and fathers of chronically sick children were more likely to have been treated for 'nerves' compared with parents of a healthy group, and mothers of chronically sick children also showed more negative affect scores. Other variables, such as social isolation or alcohol problems did not distinguish between the groups. Neither was there any difference in the incidence of single parent families. The overall picture to be drawn from this study is of much less dysfunction than is typically concluded from smaller- scale, clinic-based samples.

In the study by Wallander *et al.* (1989), there was considerable variability in the degree of ill-health reported by mothers, which although occasionally severe, hardly ever reached clinical levels of maladjustment. Such variability suggests that mothers' responses may be aggravated, or in some circumstances, buffered by, other variables. It is also possible that, for some women, the practical demands of treatments serve a purpose in enabling them to feel some control over the course of the illness as well as leaving less time in which to brood and worry over the child's condition. For mothers of dying children, opportunities to participate in simple nursing care can do much to relieve the stress that is inevitably experienced at this time. After the child's death, women who nursed their child can look back with confidence that the child was always as comfortable as possible and knowing that the child died with family rather than strangers. In the same way, joining self-help groups and becoming active in organising public sympathy and support can help reduce feelings of helplessness and inadequacy.

In attempting to account for the processes underlying mothers' adjustment to their child's illness, Wallander *et al.* (1989) identified sets of *risk* and *resistance* variables. These included:

- *intra-personal variables* (severity and functional dependence associated with the disease, temperament and coping-style of the child);

- *interpersonal variables* (temperament and coping style of the mother) and

- *social-cognitive variables* (marital and family functioning, socio-economic status, family size and service utilization). (See table 6.1).

These variables are hypothesised to be inter-dependent and reciprocal in nature. For example, *intra-personal* variables include characteristics of the disease and the child. Differences in treatment demands have been discussed previously (see Chapter 1). Less tangible variables are associated with the child. There may be differences in difficulties experienced in administering treatment in so far as children themselves differ in their easiness and preparedness to cooperate. Those who are happy with regular schedules and routines may find it easier to accommodate to the diabetic regimen than those who prefer a less organised life-style.

Inter-personal variables including temperament and coping style, are likely to influence mothers' ability to elicit social support from others, or determine how professional help (such as social services) are used to the utmost advantage. One mother of a child dying from cancer described how friends and relations were initially anxious about how to behave, and would make excuses about why they could not visit the child in hospital. She would not accept any excuses, feeling it was important for the child to have visitors so that she did not feel isolated, or suspect how serious her condition was. This mother described how she would collect people and take them herself to the hospital. Although friends had their own reasons for withdrawing support when they could not cope with the imminence of the child's death, the mother was able (through considerable determination) to ensure that some support continued until the child's death. *Social-cognitive* variables, such as family size, or socio-economic status, may also influence mothers' perceptions of the severity and restrictions associated with the child's condition.

Table 6.1. A conceptual model of predictors of adjustment in mothers of sick or handicapped children (from Varni & Wallander 1988)

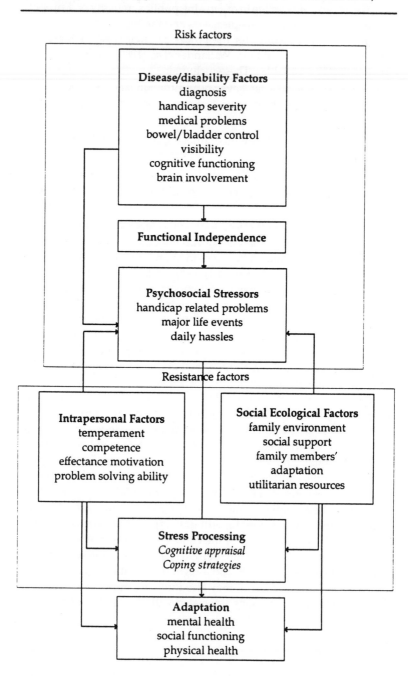

The model further assumes that families of a child with chronic disease are confronted by an increased number of potentially stressful situations; these being 'problematic situations requiring a solution or some decision-making process for appropriate action' (Varni & Wallander 1988). The way in which these stressors are dealt with is dependent on personal competence. This model does not make the assumption that the presence of a child with chronic disease in the family is necessarily associated with maladjustment. Instead, it places considerable emphasis on adaptation and resourcefulness in mothers' efforts to cope. This emphasis is reflected in several other recent models which also attempt to account for child and family behaviour in chronic disease (Perrin & MacLean 1987).

Recent theoretical models are essentially 'multivariate' in nature; that is, they acknowledge that adjustment is multiply determined. As such, they constitute a considerable advance over the more traditional, or linear models, which were based on the assumption that chronic disease was necessarily and inevitably associated with maladjustment or problems. While these recent models offer relatively comprehensive listings of variables that may potentially contribute to psychological outcome, they are often less specific about the underlying processes involved. For example, family size may act as a 'buffer'. Anxiety about the sick child may be relatively contained where there are a number of other children in the family, simply because parents have many other commitments. Alternatively, parents with large families may feel under disproportionately greater stress, as the demands involved in caring for other children restrict the time available to care for the sick child. Thus, it is unclear how family size contributes to adjustment. Similar problems arise in interpreting the contribution of other variables. In discussing how they coped with leukemia in their child, one couple said that they had always managed well, because they had previously coped with the death of one of their own parents. They felt that what they had learned practically (in organising the funeral) and emotionally (in accepting the death) prepared them for the task of caring for their child. Another couple, explaining why they had taken the diagnosis in their child so badly, attributed this partly to the recent death of one of their parents, arguing that so much stress in rapid succession had drained their resources and left them unable to respond appropriately. In any model of adjustment, it is therefore essential to build in some notion of perceived or appraised stress, in order to account for the differential impact of apparently similar experiences.

From methodological and theoretical perspectives, the dimension that is most frequently neglected is time. In most of the research reported, it is common simply to describe the sample in terms of time since diagnosis, although the analysis does not always take the variable into account. Yet it is clear that mothers' response to the child's disease is very much a dynamic phenomenon; the despair that is so usually expressed on diagnosis is much tempered by the passage of time. Diseases themselves vary greatly in stability. In conditions such as arthritis or haemophilia, mothers are able to feel relatively confident about the course of the disease; in others, especially cancer or renal disease, the future is less certain. While coping with the effects of the disease, families experience many other stresses and life-changes, and these have a significant impact on mothers' responses. Some confusion about the impact of childrens' chronic disease on mothers' mental health is the result of a failure to consider changes in the emotional impact over the course of a disease.

Factors which affect mothers' mental health
Time since diagnosis
The diagnosis of any chronic condition in the child is likely to be associated with degrees of distress and psychological ill-health for both mothers and fathers. During the initial period, parents have to come to terms with the knowledge that a previously healthy child has a chronic illness, for which there is no available cure. Often, because of the child's age or ill-health on diagnosis, parents may be more aware of the long-term implications of the disease and anxious about the consequences for the child. Aside from the emotional issues, parents must take on many aspects of daily care, while at the same time attending to the everyday needs of other children in the family and fulfilling work commitments. It would therefore not be surprising to find that the period immediately following diagnosis was particularly critical, and this is reflected in the results of much research. For example, Vandvik and Eckblad (1991) found that 50 per cent of mothers of a child with newly diagnosed rheumatic disease evidenced psychiatric levels of distress. Similarly, Koski (1969) reported that parents responded in terms of bewilderment, shock, anxiety, fear, insomnia, depression and guilt to the diagnosis of diabetes in their child. Depression and overall distress were reported in mothers who were told of diabetes in their child (Kovacs *et al.* 1985). About one in four mothers coped by 'mourning'; mentally rehearsing and preparing themselves for the possibility of the child's death. Responses typically were not influenced by the age of the child and consisted of feeling tired, worried and irritable. Mild anxiety and distress in the form of feeling tense and vulnerable, head-aches and memory problems were also reported. However, in this latter study, these emotional reactions dissipitated during the first year of treatment.

While high levels of distress are not surprising in the period immediately following diagnosis, there are several reasons to suppose that responses may moderate over time. Particularly in a condition such as diabetes, parents may realise that many aspects of life are less compromised than they initially feared. Once past the initial diagnosis, children are able to return to school as well as take part in almost all normal age-related activities. The treatment, which may appear difficult and highly demanding at first, turns out to be less of a hassle than expected. In addition, parents may find that other work and family commitments are no different from before, and need to be considered. Over time, the emotional trauma, while never receding, certainly changes.

Kovacs *et al.* (1990) studied mothers of children with diabetes from diagnosis for a period of six years. On diagnosis, the children were aged between 8 and 13 years. Mothers completed measures of depression (Beck 1967) and coping with diabetes, including assessments of the extent to which specific aspects of diabetes (for example, insulin reactions or the implications of diabetes for the child's life) bother or upset the parent, and how difficult various aspects of treatment (for example, injections, dietary restrictions) were found to be. Mothers' responses on these scales were considered in relation to measures of their child's depression and anxiety, as well as indices of the disease process, including duration, metabolic control and number of hospitalizations.

Although mothers appeared less distressed 6-9 months following diagnosis (Kovacs *et al.* 1985), levels of depression then increased again over the six-year follow-up. On diagnosis, 17 per cent of the sample could be categorized as moderately or severely depressed (Scores 16); the proportion decreased to 9 per cent at the end of the six-year period. Levels of depression at the end of the study period were predicted best from levels of depression and overall distress on diagnosis. Mothers' emotional distress was also related to the degree to which they found management of the disease to be bothersome, but not to children's anxiety or depression or variables which reflect the course of the disease, including the number of hospitalisations or metabolic control.

Mothers of higher socio-economic status exhibited more depression than other mothers. It may be that these mothers were also more educated and as such more aware of the potential complications and limitations that diabetes might impose on their children. Kovacs *et al.* (1990), suggested that for mothers of lower socio-economic status, the demands of diabetes management were not so much greater or distinguishable from other aspects of deprivation.

The lack of a comparison group imposes some restrictions on the interpretation of these data, in that it is not clear if mothers of children with other chronic conditions would respond in the same way as mothers of children with diabetes. Indeed, in conditions where the child's health is less stable, it is probable that mothers' trauma would definitely increase over time.

Leukemia is the classic example of a condition in which the child's health can change markedly over time. Although children may be considered medically cured if they survive for five years or more after all treatment ends, parents may always experience a degree of unease about the child's health. Concerns heighten on birthdays or significant anniversaries (the day the child was diagnosed), or if the child seems unwell, even if this is really only a minor everyday cold. Fear of recurrence or secondary cancers can mean that parents are never truly free from concern about the child's health.

'Other mothers worry about their child being run over or having some kind of accident. For me, there are all those worries and others about the illness, and risk of secondaries and side-effects of drugs as well' (Mother of 4 year old treated for leukemia).

Kupst and her colleagues (Kupst & Schulman 1980; Kupst et al. 1982; Kupst 1992) have traced family coping with childhood leukemia over a ten year period. Immediately after diagnosis, most families appeared to cope well, to relate well with staff, and to accept the diagnosis intellectually, if not emotionally. One third of mothers were highly anxious throughout the first year, and both parents showed wide fluctuations in mood and behaviour. At the end of the first year, most families were trying to adopt a policy of 'open communication', were employing a day-to-day orientation to life, were optimistic, and tried to treat their children as normally as possible. Two years after diagnosis, some 16 per cent of mothers and fathers were discussing the problems openly, but the same number were refusing to discuss the illness at all. Most parents reported that they themselves had experienced significant changes in their own behaviour and attitudes since the diagnosis. Over half reported that they felt more positive; but 10 per cent reported a deterioration in family relationships and inability to make long term plans. Forty per cent of families were involved in leukemia related activities, such as fund-raising. In retrospect, parents reported that the most difficult times were around diagnosis, and during painful treatments.

Age of the child

Mothers of preschool children in general appear more distressed than mothers of older children and this appears to be aggravated where the child has a chronic condition. Walker, Ford and Donald (1987) compared mothers of children with cystic fibrosis with mothers of healthy controls. Although mothers of those with cystic fibrosis did not report more daily stress, or feelings of less competence associated with being parents, those with preschoolers or adolescents were relatively more distressed than mothers of healthy children of comparable age. Such a differential was not found in comparisons with other age-groups. Caring for children in either the preschool or adolescent age- group is associated with special difficulties, and these may well be aggravated when the child is also chronically sick. Findings such as these highlight the need to be aware of the developmental implications of chronic disease so that interventions can be targeted during those periods of most need.

Disease characteristics
Since there have been very few comparative studies to assess the mental health of mothers depending on their child's particular disease, there are few real indications that some diseases are associated with more distress than others. Cummings, Bayley and Rie (1966) compared mothers of 60 mentally retarded children, 60 children with neuroses, 60 with chronic diseases (including rheumatic fever, diabetes and cystic fibrosis) and 60 healthy children. Mothers of those with chronic diseases reported lower self-esteem and less enjoyment of their children than mothers of healthy or mentally retarded children. Breslau, Staruch and Mortimer (1982) compared mothers of 77 children with cystic fibrosis, 118 with cerebral palsy, 82 with spina bifida and 92 with a range of conditions with 456 mothers of healthy controls. Although the mothers of the chronically ill groups reported more anxiety and depression, there was no difference between mothers depending on the child's particular condition.

Wallander *et al.* (1989) studied 50 mothers of children aged between 6 and 11 years who were suffering from spina bifida or cerebral palsy. In general, these mothers reported more physical and mental health complaints than mothers of healthy children, but these were not related to the severity of the child's condition or the amount of practical care the mothers were required to give.

One of the more comprehensive studies directed at the question of mothers' mental health in relation to the caretaking demands of specific conditions was reported by Jessop, Reissman and Stein (1988). The study involved 219 children, with diagnoses of asthma, seizure disorders, haemoglobinopathy, congenital heart disease, malignancies, diabetes, and a variety of congenital abnormalities. Two measures of health status were derived. The first, the Clinician's Overall Burden Index (COBI) included five dimensions:

1. Medical/nursing tasks that the parent had to perform;

2. Disruption in family routines created by these demands;

3. Deficits in the child requiring compensatory parent behaviour;

4. Dependency in a child who cannot perform age-appropriate activities, and

5. The psychological burden imposed by the child's prognosis.

Clinicians rated the extent to which a disease imposed demands on a family in the above areas in comparison with raising a healthy child of the same age. A second measure, the Functional Status Measure, was concerned with the morbidity status of the child from the perspective of the mother. The focus of the measure was the extent to which mothers saw the disease as affecting the child's capacity to perform age-appropriate roles and tasks. Daily functioning in the areas of communication, mobility, mood, eating, sleep, energy and toileting were assessed, as well as general indices of leisure, work and rest. behaviours were assessed in relation to three situations; home, neighbourhood and school. Mothers' mental health was assessed using a 29-item Psychiatric Symptom Index (Ilfield, 1976).

Mothers' mental health was related to the Functional Status Measure (i.e. her assessments of the impact of the disease), but not at all to ratings derived from the Clinician's Overall Burden Index. Jessop, Riessman and Stein (1988) argue that the impact of chronic disease can only be understood within the larger context in which families function. Unlike much work in this area, the sample of mothers involved in this study were drawn from an underpriviledged, inner-city population, who were subject to considerable stress in addition to the child's disease. (For example, 55% received public assistance; 40% were married, the rest divorced or single, and 60% were Hispanic, 27% Black and 13% of other races). At least under these circumstances, the match between clinicians' estimates of the impact of chronic disease bore little relationship to the impact assessed by the mother. The presence of other stressors in the family, poor physical health of the mother, and the absence of a confidant, increased womens' susceptibility to mental health problems.

Outside employment

Caring for a child with a chronic disease often decreases mothers' opportunities to work outside the home. The daily demands of treatment managements, need for regular clinic attendances, and increased school absences, mean that it is very difficult for mothers to take on full-time employment (Breslau, Staruch & Mortimer 1982; Cowen *et al.* 1985; Hauenstein 1987; Wasilewski *et al.* 1988) and many tend to give up employment altogether (Meyerowitz & Kaplan 1967; Tiller, Ekert & Rickards 1977). There are increased expenses incurred as a result of the disease (in relation to travel costs, or special foods or equipment). Even where medical insurance covers the cost of medication and hospitalisation, parents continue to experience considerable financial burden

(Kalnins, Churchill & Terry 1980). This means that, despite the considerable practical difficulties, many women find it necessary to work outside the home if at all possible. Women are also influenced by modern cultural norms emphasising individualistic values, personal freedom and higher status assigned to work outside, rather than within the family home. Increasingly, the norms are for women, even those with young children, to work outside the home, and many are keen to do so.

Yet it is particularly difficult for those with a chronically sick child to work in this way. Hauenstein (1987) reported that 10 of a sample of 14 mothers of chronically ill children were not employed outside the home, whereas all but one of 11 mothers of well children were. Walker, Ortiz-Valdes and Newbrough (1989) studied 95 mothers of children with one of three conditions: cystic fibrosis, diabetes, or mental retardation and compared them with mothers of healthy children. Irrespective of the condition and socio-economic status, women employed outside the home were less depressed than those who remained at home. However, women who were employed identified particular crises periods, such as when the child was ill, when they experienced extremely high levels of distress, as a result of trying to balance the separate demands of work and the family. The degree of stress at these crises times was considerable, and should not be underestimated. However, at other times, it seemed that the social contacts made at work, and opportunities to be involved in activities other than the care of the sick child, may act as some kind of buffer to protect women from very high levels of distress.

The impact of maternal employment on her mental health is ultimately dependent on the family situation, and intimately bound up with the reason for her employment. Breslau and Marshall (1985) found that in middle-class families, a child with chronic disease reduced the probability that mothers would work outside the home. In contrast, in poorer or one-parent families, the presence of a child with chronic disease increased the probability that mothers would seek outside employment. The extent to which mothers benefit psychologically from employment outside the home and are buffered against domestic stress is also dependent on her perception of the necessity of working and implicit rewards in the work environment.

It should not be concluded from this research that mothers of chronically ill children should take on outside employment. Decisions about working or not need to take into account many considerations and a desire to have more time available to spend with the child may feel much more right for many women.

Fathers' responses to chronic disease in their child

Issues relating to fathers' role in the family are increasingly discussed. More women now work outside the home, men work shorter hours and there has been a slow blurring of traditional sex-role boundaries. Many men need and want to be more involved in the care and up-bringing of their children (Baruch & Barnett 1986). The need for them to be involved is perhaps especially acute where a child is chronically ill.

Fathers do seem to respond differently from mothers to the diagnosis of chronic disease in their child. The stereotypic account of the father is one of stoicism and minimal involvement, bordering on detachment. This view has developed from observations that fathers tend to be less involved in interactions with medical staff; it is invariably mothers who bring the child, at least to routine medical appointments. The view is further corroborated from research concerned with differences between men and women in their preferred coping styles. Women are more likely to seek social support and attempt to cope by talking through their problems compared with men (Hauenstein 1987; Kazak, Reber & Carter 1988). This difference in coping style can also (perhaps erroneously) be interpreted as evidence that men are less involved or concerned about their child compared with mothers.

Following from this paternal absence in the clinic, is his non-availability to take part in research. Consequently, our understanding of how fathers respond is based on very little systematic study. As described above, fathers appear to be less likely to suffer from mental ill-health than mothers; they are less likely to respond by showing increased signs of depression and anxiety; they understand less about the disease, and they are less involved in everyday practical care. Much work points to emotional detachment in fathers of chronically sick children (Cowen *et al.* 1985; Steinhauer, Mushin & Rae-Grant 1983). According to Cummings (1976) and Tavormina *et al.* (1976), fathers of chronically ill children enjoy them less and find parenting less rewarding than fathers of healthy children. More recently, however, Eiser *et al.* (1991a) found no differences of this kind between fathers of preschool children with asthma and fathers of healthy controls.

Although there have been few studies which have directly compared mothers and fathers in terms of their emotional responses to the child's condition, there is some empirical evidence that fathers really are less adversely affected than mothers. Walker, Thomas and Russell (1971) found that only 19 out of 106 (18%) mothers of children with spina bifida reported 'feeling well' compared with 40 of 86 (46%) of fathers. In the same sample, 56 mothers reported being tired, worried or depressed, compared with only 8 fathers. In a related study involving mothers and fathers of children with leukemia (McCarthy 1975), 33 per cent of mothers and 12 per cent of fathers were found to have been prescribed anti-depressants or sleeping tablets. Results from the Ontario Child Health Study (Cadman *et al.* 1991) suggest that both mothers and fathers of chronically sick and disabled children show increased mental health problems over a normal population, although the extent of the problem is greater for mothers compared with fathers.

Yet it would be wrong to conclude that mothers made all the sacrifices while fathers made no concessions at all. While mothers of chronically ill children may be less likely to take up any kind of outside employment, fathers may have to turn down promotion, or may not be considered for promotion, especially where the child's disease limits the family's mobility (Hauenstein 1987; McKeever 1983). Many families are unhappy to move from specified areas, since they feel uncertain about the kind of care they might be offered. Tiller, Ekert & Rickards (1977) found that fathers' work and promotion opportunities were very limited, especially where they were unwilling to spend time away from the rest of the family because of the child's illness.

While fathers may not play a leading role in caring for the sick child, the evidence suggests they play a crucial supporting role. McKeever (1981) found that fathers were as distressed as mothers about their child's illness, but they interpreted their role to be in supporting their wives. These fathers acknowledged that they had less contact with hospitals compared with mothers, but felt at the same time that they were as involved in childcare at home. Klein and Simmons (1979), studying the impact of chronic renal disease on families, found that, as mothers spent longer in care and treatment of the sick child, fathers increased their contribution to more general chores and care of well children. Rarely, though, did they provide more direct help with the sick child. Most research points to the fact that fathers may not do so much in practical terms, but their presence and support is vital in buffering the effects of childhood chronic disease on mothers' mental health (Nagy & Ungerer 1990), and in facilitating her care-giving and coping (Friedrich 1979).

Fathers' family role

Our understanding of the role played by fathers in families of chronically sick children is limited because in large part, research has relied on mothers' reports of the impact of the disease on fathers, and her perceptions of his attitudes and coping responses. This type of research has yielded some inconsistent results, in that although most research suggests that mothers are more adversely affected, a proportion suggests that some fathers feel the impact of the child's condition very acutely. Although mothers often report that their husband's role is less in terms of direct, tangible help, and more generally supportive, it is not clear that fathers themselves see the situation in exactly the same way. Only a handful of studies have involved both mothers and fathers, and thus give insight into how fathers themselves perceive the child's illness, and their role in care.

Nagy and Ungerer (1990) interviewed 37 mothers and fathers of 42 children with cystic fibrosis. The results suggest that parents' mental health is dependent on their relationship, but the processes whereby this is achieved differs. Although parents did not differ in their perceptions of the stresses involved in rearing a child with cystic fibrosis, mothers showed poorer mental health than fathers. However, within the sample of fathers, mental health was inversely related to their perceptions of the total number of stresses involved. It was also related to mothers' perceptions of the difficulties involved in caring for the child; i.e. fathers' mental health was worse where mothers reported higher levels of disease-related stresses.

Mothers who received considerable social support from their husbands reported better mental health. However, the degree to which mothers saw their husbands to be supportive was not related to the actual amount of care or help that fathers offered. Rather, mothers' mental health was related to the extent to which fathers believed it to be important that they were involved in child-care. 'It appears that it is not what fathers actually do for mothers that is important for mothers' mental health, but rather, it is the value which fathers attach to child-rearing activities that is important to mothers' mental health' (Nagy & Ungerer 1990, p.152).

Differences between mothers and fathers in their perceptions of, and behaviour towards, sick children

Social support

'People were great at first. My mother-in-law came and looked after the other children. My sister, well, we've never been that close, but she would come over whenever we asked her. My firm was very good; 5 weeks off on full pay. But everyone has their own lives to lead; there's a limit to what they can do. We don't really see anyone anymore'. (Father of 10-year-old girl with cancer)

Differences between mothers and fathers in their stress responses to having a child with chronic disease, (i.e. that mothers generally show more depression, anxiety and general concern than fathers), parallel findings in other areas suggesting that women respond more emotionally to any crisis compared with men. A number of alternative models have been put forward to account for the processes underlying differential responses of men and women to stress (Hobfoll 1991). The *exposure* hypothesis explains the finding simply in terms of greater exposure to stress. However, since controlling the number of events to which men and women are exposed does not reduce or eliminate gender differences (Thoits 1987), what is considered crucial may be exposure to events over which one feels no personal control. The *role overload* model suggests that women confront multiple and lower status role stressors, whereas men confront higher status and more focussed stressors related to work (Vanfossen 1986). In the context of childhood disease, it is expected that women have greater responsibility than men for the care of the sick child. A third model attributes womens' greater depression to *poverty of personal resources*. It may be that women are not socialized in a way that develops key personal resources and they are consequently more vulnerable to mental ill-health.

Hobfoll (1991) summarizes three hypotheses about why social support may be related to increased depression in women. The first emphasises that social support is associated with costs as well as benefits. The costs include mutual sharing of problems, time out from other activities, and sometimes an awareness that the efforts put into supporting others are not appreciated. Thus, a negative consequence of interaction with others may be an increased burden for women, in that they are forced to share the worries and concerns of others; thus increasing their own burden rather than easing it.

Second, since women have to rely on men for support, they receive poorer quality of support than men, who have the advantage of receiving more considered support from women. In support of this argument, both men and women tend to report that they prefer the company of women, perhaps because women are socialized to be more nurturant (Hobfoll 1986). The result is that women benefit less from spouse support than men. Third, Doyle (1983) suggests that men are less comfortable than women about seeking help and are therefore less likely to perceive the effects of social support positively. This argument implies that women are more likely to benefit from social support than men, either because they feel more comfortable in requesting help, or because they are more skilled in using social support.

In his own work, Hobfoll (1991) interviewed 107 women and 28 men on admission of their child to hospital and again one year later. The children were drawn from a variety of settings; (1) a day care unit for non-serious illnesses; (2) an asthma out-patient clinic; (3) a neurological out-patient clinic and (4) an in-patient ward. First, the data suggest that both men and women show increases in depression over the course of the child's illness. Second, support for the *role-overload* model was found in that women were more likely than men to accompany the sick child to clinic, miss work and deal with medical staff. Men particularly avoided what became the routine care of accompanying a chronically sick child to hospital.

> 'Such role overload could explain why mothers were higher than fathers in depression both during crisis and everyday circumstances, as they have less choice in what they must confront and may be taking up the slack left over from their husband's picking and choosing when to help with family responsibilities. This finding was so striking that there was no need for statistical analysis. Where chronic illnesses confronted children, women alone were charged with care-taking responsibilities. This should not be construed to mean that men are forcing this role on women, but that socialization engenders such division of labour, such that both men and women consider these role divisions to be natural. Indeed, if men are not socialized to be nurturant, they are likely not to be helpful to the child, if they were to accompany the child. Also, although the illness of a child affects both parents, women may define their role as more interventionist than men and may feel more responsible for childrens' health' (Hobfoll 1991, p.106).

Third, there was some support for the *stress-contagion* hypothesis. Men were found to withdraw socially from others, thus not adding to their own distress through contagion with others' stresses.

Knowledge and optimism

Mothers and fathers also differ in their understanding of the child's condition and their beliefs about the prognosis and limitations. These differences have implications for their perceptions of, and behaviour toward the child, as well as acting as potential causes of disagreements between them. Mothers tend to understand more about the medical condition than fathers. This has been shown in couples with a child with cystic fibrosis (Nolan *et al.* 1986) and diabetes (Collier & Etzwiler 1971; Johnson *et al.* 1982).

Mothers seem to be less optimistic than fathers about the child's prognosis, and more likely to confess to future anxieties and concerns. Banion, Miles and Carter (1983) reported that mothers of children with diabetes were especially likely to be concerned about the possibility of future complications compared with fathers. Mulhern, Crisco and Camitta (1981) found that both mothers and fathers of children with leukemia were more optimistic about their child's survival compared with physicians, but fathers and children themselves were more optimistic than mothers. Affleck, Tennen and Rowe (1990) interviewed mothers and fathers following the discharge of their newborn baby from an intensive care unit. Parents expressed few concerns about their child's long-term prognosis, but mothers were more likely than fathers to be anxious about the possibility that the child would be mentally retarded.

In assessing issues such as the severity of their child's condition, or likelihood of survival, parents may have available a variety of information. In leukemia, for instance, various presenting features, such as the size of the child's spleen or number of white cells are taken as broad indicators of prognosis by medical staff. Whether or not this is communicated to, or understood by parents, would depend on the policies of the hospital, attitudes of staff and how well this very complex information is put across. Some of mothers' pessimism may emanate from their increased interaction with medical staff compared with fathers and consequent greater understanding of the medical condition. Other differences between parents may result from differential perceptions of the limitations imposed on the child by the condition.

CHAPTER 7

Impact of Chronic Disease on Parents and Relationships with their Children

Relationships between parents

Looking after a child with a chronic disease makes a significant impact on the level of practical and emotional stresses of the whole family. These stresses have many consequences for the parents' relationship with each other. Not only do they have to deal with all the routine difficulties shared by parents of young children everywhere, but they also have to acknowledge that their son or daughter may have a limited life-expectancy and/or be subject to many painful experiences and reduced opportunities.

Willis, Elliot and Jay (1982) summarised a number of ways in which the stress of childhood chronic disease can undermine the parental relationship. First, there are demands related to the disease and its treatment. Over and above the very practical burdens, such as giving the child medication or preparing a special diet, is the constant need for greater vigilance with regard to many aspects of the child's life. Thus, it is not just a question of giving the child medication, but often the decision needs to be taken as to whether or not medication is appropriate given the specific circumstances. For example, parents of children with asthma often report that they are in a constant state of 'red alert' and unable to relax, even at times when the asthma seems to be under relatively good control (Wasilewski et al. 1988). They must decide if a wheeze is minor and will clear itself, or if some remedial action should be taken to prevent a more major asthma attack. Arguments can be caused where one parent is naturally cautious and prefers to medicate the child at the first sign of a symptom, and the other favours a more wait and see approach.

Whatever the family is doing, the knowledge that the child might have an attack is always in the back of parents' minds. Regardless of the specific condition, parents inevitably have to make a series of complex judgments about the meaning of symptoms and efficacy of treatment, often in situations where they have less than ideal information. Judgments about whether or not the child is genuinely ill, or 'pretending' need to be made almost on a daily basis (Gonder-Frederick, Clarke & Snyder 1987).

Second, parents' relationships can be strained by the demands of care-taking. This can create friction between parents as to who bears the major responsibility, and severely limit the amount of time that is then available for recreation, each other, or other children in the family.

Third, often as a consequence of heightened care-taking demands, parents have to work hard to maintain family integrity; finding time for other children and working out ways of functioning as a family. Healthy siblings may resent the time parents spend with sick children, and often complain about the lack of attention given to them.

Fourth, parents have to find a way to ensure financial stability. Chronic disease may involve a family in considerable expenses which are not incurred by families of healthy children. Travel to clinics and hospitals, baby-sitting for other children, foods for special diets or presents to cheer the child up, can all contribute a real strain to financial resources. These costs are in addition to the more major limitation imposed by the restrictions on one or other parent working as much as they would like, or for some families, the costs of the treatment itself.

Given the number of difficulties that confront parents in these situations, it is hardly surprising that it is frequently suggested that the divorce rate is higher than in the general population. Even where families remain intact it seems that the quality of parents' relationships with each other is the first to suffer. For example, Donnelly, Donnelly and Thong (1987) reported that 34 per cent of families of children with asthma felt that the child's disease had an adverse effect on the parents' relationship with each other. Yet asthma can be a relatively mild condition, which imposes few long-term restrictions on the child's mobility or opportunities to participate in age-appropriate activities. Neither does it impose unreasonable care-taking demands on parents. Diseases which are associated with these limitations may be expected to compromise the quality of parent's relationships more routinely.

Even so, those who do divorce only rarely report the child's disease to be a central, or even contributory factor. Martin (1975) reported that few families specifically cited the child's disease as a reason for their divorce. Of three divorces in a sample of 120 families with a child with spina bifida, (Hare et al. 1966) all implicated the child's condition as being the main cause. Sometimes differences between parents in their general attitudes to life can be contained until a crisis acts to polarise their responses. So for a long time it may not matter if one parent is naturally cautious and the other is more prepared to take risks. Real conflicts only occur when the parents are confronted by the threats of the illness. In these cases, there may be conflicts specifically about the treatment and the way it is handled. In addition, one parent can find that they no longer find the partner's general attitudes tolerable at all.

Other work suggests that the disease, and attempts to deal with it, can bring families closer together (Barbarin *et al.* 1985; Koocher & O'Malley 1981; Vance *et al.* 1981). In summarising research before 1980, Kalnins (1983) reported that between 20 to 50 per cent of parents reported a strengthening of their marriage, following the diagnosis of the child's disease. Certainly, this more cohesive approach seems to characterise parents' initial response to diagnosis. Work reviewed in the following section points to the probability of divorce and marital dissatisfaction increasing with the length of time since diagnosis and any deterioration in the child's health.

Prevalence of divorce in couples with a child with chronic disease

Divorce rates in couples with a child with chronic disease have been compared with national or state norms, or across different disease groups. In studies of families with a child with cystic fibrosis, (Allan, Townley & Phelan 1974); cancer, (Lansky *et al.* 1978); muscular dystrophy (Buchanan *et al.* 1979); spina bifida (Freeston 1971); renal disease (Vance *et al.* 1981) and congenital heart disease (Silbert, Newburger & Fyler 1982), divorce rates were comparable to those in the general population or matched controls. Results from the Ontario Child Health Study, which included children with a range of chronic and disabling conditions, found no increase in single parent families in the total group compared with population controls (Cadman *et al.* 1991).

Other studies have shown some increases in divorce rates. Tew, Payne and Laurence (1974) reported twice as many divorces in families with a child with spina bifida compared with a normal sample. These data were collected over a nine-year period following diagnosis. While it is possible that spina bifida creates particular practical problems which make couples more vulnerable to divorce, it is also possible that these results reflect an increasing vulnerability with the longer the time involved. (The previous studies cited did not take into account any relationship between divorce vulnerability and the length of time the child was ill). Further evidence that couples with a child with spina bifida may be especially vulnerable comes from two other studies. Martin (1975) reported that divorce rates in a clinic population of spina bifida families was higher than either a normal control group or couples having a child with diabetes. Kazak and Wilcox (1984) also reported an increased incidence of divorce among couples with a child with spina bifida compared with a matched sample with healthy children.

These inconsistent research findings can be partly attributed to methodological problems in research design, particularly to differences between studies in selection of samples and sample size (Kalnins 1983). The most common selection procedure involves contacting families whose child was born or diagnosed within a specified period of time. Divorce rates for these groups are then compared against census statistics. However, since census statistics represent divorce rates in a particular year and do not provide information about changes in rate over a period of time, they are not comparable with divorce rates for families of chronically sick children, which are usually based on cumulative rates. This procedure is likely to yield apparently elevated divorce rates for the families of sick children.

More acceptable sampling procedures involve random selection, since this method is less likely to result in bias from refusal by some families to participate. Families with known social or emotional difficulties are especially likely to refuse to participate in research.

In addition to problems of sample selection, Kalnins (1983) notes that difficulties arise because of differences in sample size. In the studies reviewed in this article, sample size varied from 13 to 214 families. A re-analysis of these data resulted in a reported negative correlation between sample size and calculated divorce rate, such that higher divorce rates were reported in studies involving fewer families. Yet even larger sample sizes are no guarantee of consistent results. Denning, Gluckson and Mohr (1976) found a divorce rate of 10.6 per cent when working with a sample of 103 families. The calculated divorce rate dropped to 6.5 per cent as the sample size was expanded to 214 families. In the studies reviewed by Kalnins (1983), it was found that the five studies involving the smallest sample sizes reported both the lowest and highest divorce rates (Stebhens & Lascari 1974; Tiller, Ekert & Rickards 1977).

Other variables have been implicated as contributing to divorce in families of chronically sick children. These include the existence of an unstable or distressed marriage prior to the diagnosis (Allan, Townley & Phelan 1974); conception of the affected child before marriage (Walker, Thomas & Russell 1971); and birth of the child within 18 months of marriage. This list is far from exhaustive, and is little more than an *ad hoc* selection of contender variables. Lack of a theoretical perspective limits appropriate selection of variables that either aggravate or minimize the probability of divorce rates in these families.

Divorce rates are a very gross indicator of family relationships. For the most part, research has been based on very small populations (most of the work reviewed above included samples of 30–60). These studies shed no light on the reasons for the divorce; neither do they give any insight as to the quality of the relationship where marriages do remain intact, despite the child's condition. Often, mothers are the only source of information, and little attention is paid to fathers' perceptions of, or satisfaction with the marriage (Sabbeth & Leventhal 1984). These authors reviewed the results from a number of different studies (seven involving parents of children with spina bifida, six involving parents of those with cystic fibrosis, four with congenital heart disease and two with cancer). Fifteen other studies involving parents of children with a number of chronic conditions were also considered. Taking all these studies together, there was no evidence of higher divorce levels than in the general population.

However, divorce statistics are only one measure of the impact of disease, and far from the most satisfactory. They reveal nothing about relationships within marriages, or the reasons why some couples choose to remain married when, under apparently similar or even more favourable situations, others choose to separate. For these reasons, it is more important to consider the quality or satisfaction that is intrinsic to a marriage, and the ease with which individuals feel comfortable and able to communicate with each other.

For many reasons, both relating to methodological problems in the way in which this research is conducted, and more theoretical issues concerned with the processes underlying marital relationships, some researchers have become increasingly concerned to describe the quality of marriages, particularly with regard to the individual partner's satisfaction with the relationship, or the degree and accuracy of communication. The quality of marital adjustment is generally assessed in relation to variables such as marital distress, intimacy, communication, decision-making and role-flexibility.

QUALITY

'Marital quality' is an elusive concept. Modern beliefs, at least in Western societies, focus on the advantages of marriage for the individuals concerned, and less, if at all, on the implications for children and extended family relationships more generally. In keeping with this view, attempts to assess marital quality have adopted one of two approaches. Some see marital quality in terms of how individuals feel about their marriages, and therefore rely on self-reports of marital satisfaction or happiness. An alternative approach emphasises the nature of the *relationship* between individuals, rather than focussing on separate feelings of the individuals involved. Criticisms of both approaches have been put forward (Fincham 1985), with the result that there appears to be little concensus among researchers as to how marital quality can best be conceptualized (Fitzpatrick 1990).

Nevertheless, much effort has been directed toward assessing the quality or satisfaction experienced by parents where a child has a chronic disease compared with the experiences of parents of healthy children. This approach is based on an implicit assumption that parents of chronically sick children are more likely to experience and report marital problems and dissatisfaction than parents of healthy children. A second approach looks at differences between parents as a function of the particular condition of the child. Both approaches are more concerned to identify difficulties experienced and make little acknowledgement of any rewards which parents may find in parenting their children, regardless of their health status. Much of the work must be criticised for focussing on difficulties, and often allowing parents few opportunities to describe family strengths or adjustments to the management of the disease. Neither do they readily allow for comparisons to be made depending on social or economic resources of the family, nor in relation to changes in experiences with childrens' age or other family situations.

In all marriages, quality is generally rated less highly in families with a preschool or teenage child, compared with families with children of middle school age or without children.

Nevertheless, with very few exceptions, studies suggest that parents of chronically sick children report considerable marital distress and dissatisfaction; these are generally greater than found in matched samples of parents of healthy children; levels of reported distress are higher among mothers than fathers, and differ somewhat as a function of disease. These conclusions have been based on studies involving parents of children with cystic fibrosis (Allan et al. 1974; Cowen et al. 1985); cancer (Heffron, Bommelaere & Masters 1976; Barbarin, Hughes & Chesler 1985; Crain, Sussman & Weil 1966); renal disease (Reynolds et al. 1988) and spina bifida (Tew et al. 1974).

Invited to take part in research concerned with the impact of chronic disease on marital functioning, it is perhaps not surprising that parents report difficulties. It is after all, what the researchers appear to be interested in, and studies are often introduced to parents with the expressed aim that 'we are trying to find out how we can best help parents look after a child with a chronic condition'. Parents would be accused of denial if they suggested that the presence of the sick child in the family made little difference to their relationship, or even enhanced it. From this point of view, the way in which chronic disease affects the parents' relationship may be investigated more systematically by considering parents' reports in relation to different conditions.

Cairns and Lansky (1980) compared the marital distress reported by parents with a child with cancer with parents of a child with haemophilia in relation to healthy controls. Sixty-eight per cent of parents of

children with cancer and 39 per cent of those with a child with haemophilia showed significant levels of marital distress, compared with only
4 per cent of couples in a normative sample. Gordon Walker and Manion
(1991) compared parents of children with cancer, cystic fibrosis, renal
disease, diabetes and muscular dystrophy. For the total sample, 43 per
cent scored as maritally distressed (as indicated by scores one standard
deviation below the mean for marital satisfaction reported by Snyder
and Regts (1982) or a score of 110 or lower on Spanier's (1976) Dyadic
Adjustment Scale. However, there were no indications that levels of
marital distress varied directly as a function of a specific disease group.

Parents' satisfaction with the quality of their marriage seems to
deteriorate with the time since diagnosis. According to data reported by
McCubbin, Cauble and Patterson (1982), couples whose child was diagnosed with cancer made more favourable ratings of their marriage on
diagnosis than three years later. This is consistent with other observations that parents' initial response to the crisis is frequently one of
cohesion and mutual support. Setbacks which jeopardise the child's
health or anticipated recovery and additional hardships encountered
very much challenge the family's ability to sustain their early optimism.

COMMUNICATION AND INTERACTION

In marriages generally, communication difficulties are the major cause
of unhappiness, so that the extent to which marriages are rated as
satisfactory or not is frequently dependent on the adequacy and success
of communication (Lewis & Spannier 1979). However, couples differ in
their definitions of 'good' communication (Fitzpatrick 1984). For some,
communication serves a purpose in enabling them to analyse and work
on their relationship (Katriel & Philipsen 1981); for others communication is used to define mutual rights and obligations (Sillars et al. 1987).
Marital communication is different from any other type of communication, in that it is founded on extensive, complex and affective knowledge
systems.

Communication in marriage is more than a mere exchange of information, in that it may be used as a basis for mutually acceptable patterns
of behaviour. In caring for a chronically sick child, parents' ability to
communicate with each other will influence the way in which they
construct a definition of the disease, its etiology and implications, their
own affective responses to it, and their ability to share practical demands
and integrate these successfully into their everyday lives. In these ways,
the function of communication goes beyond that involved in other
marriages. For this reason, it is inappropriate to assess communication
in couples with a sick child in comparison with couples with a healthy
child. While the demands and purposes of communication may overlap,

the dimensions that couples perceive to be most central may be substantially different.

Very little empirical work has systematically considered the impact of a child with chronic disease on marital communication. However, a major source of conflict is likely to be the extent to which the burden of caring for the child is shared (or perceived to be shared), both at a practical level (sharing child-care and treatment demands) and more emotionally, in terms of being able to discuss responses and feelings about the illness. A number of studies suggest that mothers especially complain that they have little time for themselves after all the treatment demands have been met. Couples with a child with cystic fibrosis complained that they had little time or energy for leisure or time alone together (Turk 1964). Similar results have been reported among families with a child with cancer, (Heffron, Bommelaere & Masters 1976; Barbarin, Hughes & Chesler 1985). In both these studies, mothers also reported that they felt very much alone in caring for the child and organising other everyday aspects of family life, often with little support from their spouses.

Communication can be especially compromised when the child has an inherited condition, for which one parent blames the other. Problems arise especially in conditions involving an inherited component, such as haemophilia or cystic fibrosis (Turk 1967), asthma (Nocon 1991) and epilepsy (Voeller & Rothenberg 1973). Even in conditions where there is no known inherited component, elements of blame can cloud parents' relationships. 'There's cancer on Joan's side, see, but none on mine. There's no-one on my side of the family who's ever had cancer; it's all on Joan's side' (Father of 16-year-old).

The influence of parents' relationships for the child's adjustment and behaviour

Research interest in the prevalence of divorce and marital conflict among parents of chronically sick children should go beyond mere reporting of incidence statistics. There is conflicting evidence about the link between the severity of the child's condition or extent of the handicap and increased probability of divorce or marital dissatisfaction. It may well be that parental conflict is a *consequence* of disproportionate stress. Of potentially greater interest and practical value, however, is the question of how parents' relationship (or lack of it) influences the course of the child's disease and acceptance of medical care and treatment by child and family.

Related work concerned with the relationship between marital problems and childrens' behaviour in general populations is of some relevance to this issue. There is substantial evidence that children living in homes characterised by parental conflict are more likely to show emotional and behavioural problems than those coming from more harmonious backgrounds (Bloch, Block & Morrison 1981). What is less clear is the aspect of parental conflict which is potentially most damaging to the child. One candidate is the exposure to parent conflict and arguments, and indeed, children do show distress when witnessing adult conflict, even where this does not directly involve their parents. A second hypothesis is that parental disharmony distorts other family relationships, resulting in destructive family alliances. Third, parental conflict may affect how one parent feels or behaves towards a child. Easterbrooks and Emde (1988) found that good marital relationships were associated with greater parenting satisfaction for fathers, but that mothers' relationships with their child were independent of their own perceived marital quality.

Chronic childhood disease has the potential to disrupt and destroy parents' relationship, but it can also serve to unite them in their efforts to care for the child and overcome the many difficulties. We know very little about the determinants of these very different courses of action. Rather than focus on descriptions of parents' relationships, we need to move toward establishing how these affect the child's coping. How is it that some families create an environment in which everyone looks on the bright side and the child seems only minimally influenced by the disease? Yet others have few resources and seem to lurch from one crisis to another. While it has often been assumed that parent's behaviour influences the child, the two are of course, mutually dependent.

Impact on everyday parenting
Following the diagnosis of chronic disease in a child, parents' immediate concerns focus on the needs to understand the practical requirements of the condition. Learning about the disease is important to enable parents to become proficient themselves in administering home treatments and integrating these new routines with other everyday activities. At this time, the child may seem very ill, and the central concern is naturally with doing everything possible to help the child's initial recovery. In dealing with the emotional concerns of the child's illness, and as a response to perceptions of the child's pain and discomfort, many parents (and grand-parents!) try hard to make the child feel special and important. This behaviour can take many forms, but is often dismissed rather derogatively in terms of 'spoiling' the child. It is tempting to buy gifts, or special foods, or turn a blind eye to previously unacceptable behaviour in order to encourage the child to 'get well'.

Problems can arise when these behaviours continue beyond the initial crisis period. Difficulties occur especially for healthy siblings, who may resent, or fail to understand, why their brother or sister receives a disproportionate number of favours, or is less likely to be punished for naughty behaviour than they are. Parents' perceptions of the child's prognosis, and their understanding of the disease and its limitations may influence many of their decisions about parenting, as well as the way in which the child responds to, and attempts to reconcile the restrictions of the disease with everyday life.

The occurrence of chronic disease is likely to challenge some deep-seated beliefs about child-rearing, including attitudes to control and discipline, and education. For example, parents who were very ambitious for their child may come to question the value of education, given that the child's future seems so compromised and uncertain. Families may also perceive the child to be very fragile and vulnerable, worrying about the rough-and- tumble of the play-ground, and trying to protect the child from the everyday infections of other children.

Parental dilemmas about child-rearing are aggravated by the ambiguous nature of much chronic disease. Although the conditions are not curable, many children look normal and do not seem so very different from before the diagnosis. This is especially true in the case of conditions with very rapid onset, such as leukemia, where parents often feel they had little warning of the impending condition. It is sometimes hard to believe that the diagnosis has been made. Parents may feel that they have had a very bad dream, and expect to wake up to find that it was a dream. The dilemma is fuelled by the medical profession, who, with the best of intentions, are at pains to point out that the child should lead 'a normal life'. *There is rarely advice, however, about what constitutes 'a normal life' or how this can most easily be achieved for a child with a chronic disease.* Life can never be 'normal' for a family with a child with a life- threatening condition.

According to many early, often clinic-based observations, parents' response to their child's chronic disease is to adopt a restrictive and over-protective parenting style. This approach grew out of the prevailing psychoanalytic models of parent behaviour, with an emphasis on parental acceptance and rejection. The basic premise is that normal parental attitudes are characterised by affection. Where parents' emotional needs have not been met, Levy (1943) argues that the result is overprotection or rejection of the child. Overprotection, characterized by prolonged infantile care through excessive control was contrasted with rejection. Parent–child interaction was initially construed in terms of other excesses of parental behaviour, including anxiety, indulgence, perfectionism and strictness. This approach dominated work untill recently.

The focus on restrictive and over-protective parenting styles is increasingly recognised as too narrow and inappropriate. Methodologically, there is a bias toward data based on mothers' reports about her own and her partners' behaviour, but little effort to validate these reports with observational data. Fathers' behaviours are inevitably inferred from mothers' reports with no attempts at substantiation. Yet the issue of how chronic disease affects parenting practice is a very real one, with implications for the child's capacity for normal social and cognitive functioning. It is therefore particularly unfortunate that research in this area has been essentially eclectic, with a rather disordered focus on individual variables, and little attempt to account for how different variables relate to each other. These difficulties stem from the lack of any cohesive theoretical framework regarding parenting generally, or specifically in accounting for parenting children with chronic disease.

Theoretical approaches to parenting

The most common theoretical principals employed have utilized concepts from Exchange or Social learning theory (Bandura 1977). Emphasis is placed on factors both internal and external to the parent–child relationship. Internal to the relationship are parents' views about the rewards and costs incurred in having children. Most adults believe that children offer certain rewards such as affection, companionship and stimulation (Hoffman & Manis 1982). In some relationships, where the child is perceived to be difficult or hard-to-manage, parents may feel that the rewards they expected from parenting are not forthcoming. Chronic disease may potentially put rewards and costs out of balance, although there has been little research concerned with the disruptive effects of chronic disease in this way.

Parenting behaviour is also likely to be affected by a variety of external factors, including parental beliefs, values and emotional state, and commitments and rewards inherent in work and other emotional relationships.

Emotional state

Depressed mothers tend to report more behaviour problems in their child, and this is particularly pronounced among mothers of boys (Lancaster, Prior & Adler 1989). There is no simple answer to the issue of whether the child's difficult behaviour causes depression in mothers, or whether depressed mothers are more likely to find their child's behaviour difficult because they are depressed and have fewer resources with which to handle everyday crises. Depression has also been associated with real deficits in parenting behaviour stemming from a loss of interest in activities and situations.

Beliefs about parenting

Extending the notion of self-efficacy to parenting (Bandura 1977), parents who believe that they have a major role to play in shaping their child's behaviour and life-choices are likely to commit themselves more to the parenting role, than those who feel that the more major influences on their child emanate from school, the culture and peers. Chronic disease may well undermine parents' beliefs in their ability to care for, or shape their child's future.

Despite the hypothesised relationship between parents' beliefs about parenting and their actual behaviour, early attempts to demonstrate the relationship were only partially successful. Two kinds of maternal beliefs were distinguished by Kochanska, Kuczynski and Radke-Yarrow (1989). These included endorsed methods of child-rearing, and affective attitudes toward the child and parenting experience. In a study of toddler-age children, they showed that endorsed methods of child-rearing predicted behaviour, but affective attitudes predicted mothers' reports of difficulties experienced. Four belief clusters were also distinguished. These included an *authoritative/democratic* pattern, an *authoritarian/restrictive* pattern, *enjoyment of the child* and *negative affect* toward the child.

> 'The authoritarian pattern of maternal beliefs was associated with maternal use of direct commands, physical enforcements, reprimands and prohibitive interventions; endorsement of the authoritative pattern was associated with the use of polite suggestions and positive incentives, and negatively related to the use of enforcements, prohibitions, and direct commands. Mothers' enjoyment of child-rearing and negative affect toward their children were more associated with childrens' cooperation and resistance than predictors of maternal control attempts' (p.56).

Subsequently, Kuczynski & Kochanska (1990) showed that the endorsement of different child-rearing beliefs when the children were toddlers predicted maternal behaviour 2–3 years later. Those who initially endorsed authoritative parenting styles were found to avoid punitive actions towards their child and allowed greater autonomy at follow-up. However, the relative contributions of these belief clusters to maternal child-rearing behaviour depended on maternal mental health. Endorsed child-rearing beliefs were more important predictors of behaviour for normal mothers, but affective attitudes were better predictors for depressed mothers. For normal mothers, there was a correspondence between their professed child-rearing beliefs and their actual behaviour, which was not found for depressed mothers.

Work and parenting values

The prevailing cultural emphases on individualistic values, concerned with individual expression, personal freedom and individual success are at odds with more traditional values involved in caring for a child (Bellah *et al.* 1985). Many women are faced with a dilemma in pursuing a career and their own personal goals, rather than placing higher value on family life. The extent to which women are committed to such individualistic values has negative implications for parenting behaviours (Greenberger & Goldberg 1988).

Methodological difficulties in assessing parent–child relationships

Choice of control population

A first methodological consideration relates to the choice of control group. Choice of children with different conditions is usually made when the concern is with specific limitations associated with a particular condition. For example, work concerned with educational attainments in children with leukemia have compared the group with children treated for solid tumors. This latter group is generally justified on the grounds that children have a life-threatening disease, undergo similar procedures and chemotherapy, but do not undergo CNS irradiation. Differences between the groups can therefore be attributed directly to a specific component of the treatment. (In fact, the groups do differ on other dimensions. Those with solid tumors undergo surgery, but generally miss less school time than those with leukemia).

A second method involves using healthy siblings as 'controls'. In these cases, families may be asked to participate in a study twice over; once with reference to the chronically sick child, and once in relation to a healthy sibling. In this way, social class and family circumstances are well controlled for, and it is assumed that any differences in the ways in which parents describe or interact with their children can be attributed to the disease. Such an assumption is in fact unfounded. There is much to suggest that parents do not respond to all children in the family in the same way. Child temperament and behaviour, birth order and spacing, have all been implicated as determinants of parent behaviour (Dunn & McGuire 1992).

A third method is to include families of healthy children, matched on some demographic factors, especially where the central issue is to identify differences between chronically sick or healthy children, and where the concern is with how well the chronically sick child can be expected to be integrated in normal situations, especially at school or work. Thus, many studies looking at educational attainments in children with cancer have compared I.Q. scores or reading achievements with 'matched' control groups of healthy children (for example, Eiser &

Lansdown 1977). The rationale for this was that if children with leukemia were cured, they should be indistinguishable from the general population in all respects. Kazak (1989) argues strongly against the practice of using healthy children and families as a 'gold standard' against which the attainments and behaviour of the sick child are assessed. The demands of chronic disease may mean that *different* standards and parenting practices are more appropriate in families where there is a sick child, compared with other families. Thus, all parents may attempt to encourage their children to eat healthily, and virtually all families report some conflicts over food and eating habits. While these conflicts do not generally reach major proportions in healthy families, concern about growth and the importance of good nutrition to help combat the disease can mean that food becomes much more a bone of contention in families with a sick child. Yet it may also be more appropriate that parents attempt to influence their child's eating behaviour, especially in diseases such as diabetes or cystic fibrosis, where attention to diet is an integral part of appropriate self-care behaviour.

Cappelli *et al.* (1989) provided convincing evidence for this, in a comparison of parenting practices in families with a child with cystic fibrosis and those with healthy children. There were no overall differences in the level of parental care and overprotection between the two groups. However, different correlates of parental care were found to be associated with good psychosocial adaptation depending on the health status of the child. In healthy children, poor psychosocial functioning was associated with lack of parental care. However, among those with cystic fibrosis, poor psychosocial functioning was associated with excessive parental overprotection. Psychosocial functioning appeared to be mediated by different parenting practices, depending on the health of the child.

Questionnaire approaches

Parents' attitudes to child-rearing are most usually assessed by questionnaire. As a means of collecting data, questionnaires are undoubtedly quick and easy to administer. They are also under increasing criticism. Holden and Edwards (1989) argued that, despite the popularity of questionnaires, they fail to relate conceptually to theoretical ideas about parenting; they have been subject to limited and barely adequate psychometric assessment; their relation to other measures of parents' beliefs or thoughts is in need of clarification, and they raise certain basic issues concerning the relationship between parents' attitudes and behaviour and parent–child interaction more generally.

For present purposes, it is pertinent to illustrate their arguments by summarising their data concerned with mothers' responses to the Parental Attitudes toward Childrearing questionnaire (Easterbrooks &

Goldberg 1984). Mothers completed the questionnaire and were then interviewed about their responses to the questions and any difficulties they had experienced with specific items. The most common problems were that: responses would be influenced by the situation; mothers had never before thought about the issue and therefore had difficulties in deciding on an answer; they were confused by the response scale; thoughts about other children interfered with their ability to make decisions exclusively about the target child, and the questions were too vague. Of particular concern with regard to assessment of parent–child interaction in chronic disease, many mothers reported that at least one item was inappropriate given the age or temperament of their child. For example, parents of two-year olds pointed to the difficulty of knowing how to respond to the following item; 'I let my child make many decisions for him/herself', since it is not clear what decisions a two-year-old can reasonably be expected to make. This inappropriateness of items is very much a problem in studies of children with chronic disease, where relatively small populations of children are generally recruited from clinics, on the basis of diagnosis rather than any other criterion variable. For example, mothers of children with asthma reported these same difficulties in responding to questionnaires about their perceptions of the childrens' self-efficacy (Schlosser & Havermans 1992). Items such as 'Decide how many puffs I take when I get an attack' were in fact appropriate across a relatively narrow age range. A related difficulty concerns situational specificity. Context is invariably unspecified in general questionnaires. So items such as 'Ask for help when I get an attack' require confirmatory responses in some situations, (for example, home) but would not be endorsed in other contexts, such as school.

Problems also arose because of the vague wording of some items. Holden and Edwards (1989) suggested that mothers can give different responses to the same item simply because of alternative interpretations. They quote the example of 'I tend to spoil my child'. This item could be given one of three different meanings. Mothers might interpret the item to mean they were being too lenient, they were giving too much attention, or they were giving too many material things. If these interpretations were made by mothers of healthy children, it is necessary to clarify how mothers of sick children understand the items, and particularly to establish if differences between mothers of healthy or chronically sick children can be attributed to differences in interpretation of items as much as to differences in actual behaviour. The question arises as to whether mothers interpret items such as this differently, depending on the health of their child. One might expect particular ambiguity on items which are concerned with highly emotive concepts such as 'spoiling' the sick child, and less to items that carry less negative connotations.

A related problem and again one with considerable implication for work with parents of chronically sick children, was found in the interpretation of the *focus* of some questions. For example, it is unclear if the focus of the following item is the mother or the child: 'I sometimes feel I am too involved with my child'. Mothers (44%) who responded in terms of their own behaviour were likely to agree with the item (mean=3.4), while those (24%) who responded from the point of view of their child and themselves agreed less (mean=2.0). The remaining mothers, thinking from their child's view alone, fell in the middle (mean=2.4). A similar analysis was conducted on the item, 'I believe physical punishment to be the best way of disciplining'; again an item of considerable interest in research concerned with parenting chronically sick children. Some mothers interpreted the item as a question about how frequently they used physical punishment. Those who made this interpretation rated it higher (mean=2.6) than those who interpreted it as both a frequency and attitude item (mean=1.3).

In summary, there are many methodological problems in questionnaires in use to assess parent–child behaviours. Some of these relate to the format and development of the questionnaires generally, and others arise from the use of the scales with different populations from those intended. Particular difficulties arise in the interpretation of data derived from questionnaires. These focus on using the same questionnaire to assess behaviour across a wide age-range, and failing to specify context. Ambiguities in wording may lead to alternative interpretations and consequently bias in obtained results.

Criticisms of current methodologies

Despite the criticisms that can be leveled at methods commonly used to assess parent–child relationships, the question of how, or if, chronic disease compromises the relationship is of considerable interest both theoretically and practically. Theoretically, there is generally an assumption that understanding parent-child relationships under a variety of circumstances can contribute to more complete perspectives on the relationship generally. Any adequate theory also needs to be able to address the question of how relationships are changed under defined circumstances. Practically, provision of appropriate support and professional services to families of chronically sick children is dependent on knowledge of the relationship and indices of vulnerability. Empirical work in this area is limited and needs to be interpreted within the context of methodological limitations described.

Empirical work on parent–child relationships in chronic disease

Despite the assumption that parents modify their expectations of sick children and adopt different discipline strategies, there is very little empirical work on the topic. What there is suggests only minor, almost trivial effects on parenting. Markova, MacDonald & Forbes (1980) found that boys with mild to moderate haemophilia were given more domestic responsibilities than healthy controls. Parents of boys with haemophilia described themselves as stricter than other parents. Walker, Ford and Donald (1987) studied parenting practices in families with a child with cystic fibrosis in relation to a control group of mothers of children drawn from a primary care clinic. There were no substantial differences between the groups in assessments of their confidence in parenting or concerns about their discipline practices. However, mothers of those with cystic fibrosis reported modifying their discipline practices depending on perceived severity of the child's condition; they were more strict when the child was well, but relaxed family rules during periods when the illness was exacerbated.

Eiser *et al.* (1991a) compared mothers and fathers of pre-school children with asthma and parents of healthy controls, in terms of reported discipline practices, perceptions of the child, and situations which were particularly stressful. Again, there were no differences between the groups in terms of reported discipline practices. Parents of those with asthma described their children as less healthy (more likely to catch colds and slow to recover from minor complaints) compared with parents of healthy children, and they also perceived a greater number of everyday situations to be stressful (e.g. going shopping, putting the child to bed).

In a related study, based on the same sample of children with asthma, small differences were noted in parenting practice as a function of the severity of the child's condition (Eiser, Eiser, Town & Tripp 1991b). There were no reported differences in parenting practices, although mildly affected children were perceived to be more difficult in certain situations compared with children with more severe asthma.

There have been a substantial number of reports implying that parents of children with cancer experience difficulties in relation to discipline and control of their child. The potentially life-threatening nature of the disease, and degree of ill-health that children can experience, either directly as a result of the condition, or less directly as a consequence of side-effects of treatment, create many parenting dilemmas. Parents may be tempted to 'spoil' the child, and experience many conflicts in dealing with the child's behaviour and demands for independence (Chesler, Paris & Barbarin 1986; Powazek *et al.* 1980; Wasserman *et al.* 1987). This view is generally endorsed by physicians, who perceive parents of children with cancer to be more protective, concerned and ineffective in discipline practices compared with how they *imagine* parents of healthy children (Davies *et al*. 1991).

In addition to obtaining the views of physicians about how they thought parents of children would behave, Davies *et al*. (1991) also elicited the views of parents themselves. Self-reports of parenting practices were obtained from mothers and fathers of 24 children with cancer and 24 healthy controls. Parents completed the Child-Rearing Practices Report (Block 1981). This consists of 91 statements assessing goals, values and attitudes toward parenting. Responses are made in terms of a seven-point scale, from 'most' to 'least' descriptive of parents' behaviour.

Both mothers and fathers of children with cancer reported greater worry about their child's health compared with parents of healthy children, and mothers of children with cancer were concerned that they were too involved with their child. Otherwise, there were few differences in reported parenting practices between the two groups of parents. Although it was found that mothers of children with cancer expressed concern that they were too involved with their children, this was in fact only one of ten items included to assess over-protectiveness. There were no differences on the other nine items. In the study described above by Holden and Edwards (1989), it should be remembered that particular difficulties were identified for mothers in the way in which items of this kind were interpreted. As in the study by Eiser *et al*. (1991) which involved children with asthma, the implications are that self-reported differences between parents of sick children and healthy controls are limited to concerns about physical health and do not generalise to other issues.

Despite the long tradition from the clinical literature that chronic childhood disease compromises normal parenting practices, the empirical work that has been conducted, (which is not extensive) does not support this view. Few differences between parents of chronically sick and healthy children have been identified, and these tend to be restricted to concerns about the physical health of chronically sick children. These are perfectly reasonable concerns, and to be expected. The lack of differences in other respects is open to a number of alternative explanations. Some of these can be attributed to methodological problems, largely described earlier (Holden & Edwards 1989). It is not clear how parents perceive the task of describing their behaviour toward their children, especially under circumstances where the focus of the study is defined in terms of 'understanding how parents look after children with chronic disease'. Given these instructions and on the understanding that the researchers have some awareness of the implications of the disease, parents may respond accordingly; i.e. taking into account the fact that the child has a chronic condition and some changes in their behaviour would be expected and appropriate. Parents of healthy children, told that they are taking part in a study concerned with parenting children with a chronic condition, may also modify their responses.

This may also be an area in which there are considerable differences between how parents report they behave, compared with what they actually do. Parents may believe that it is important to treat sick children as normal, but fail to achieve this in practice. The relationship between parental beliefs about child-rearing and their actual behaviour has been discussed in the context of normal parent child relations (Goodnow 1988). She argues that parental beliefs, even if not closely related to behaviour, are important in guiding parents and shaping their attitudes to child care. Kochanska, Kuczynski and Radke-Yarrow (1989) demonstrated some relationships between maternal beliefs about child-rearing and observed behaviour, at least among mothers of 2–3 year old children. Unfortunately, very few observational studies have been conducted to investigate parent child behaviour where the child has a chronic disease.

Observational work involving mother–child and father–child relationships is generally limited to parents of young infants rather than older children, and to mother–child rather than father–child interaction (Goldberg *et al.* 1990). This work is described in detail in Chapter 2, and suggests that attachment is not seriously compromised in many parents of children with these conditions, although the development of attachment does not necessarily follow the same pattern as among healthy children and their parents.

There are some implications in the work reviewed so far that different processes underly parenting behaviour and decision-making dependent on the health status of the child. Lack of awareness of these differences, and a tendency to rely on measures of parenting developed to study healthy (or psychiatrically disturbed) parent–child relationships, limits understanding of the processes involved. Recent work which emphasises differences *within* a sample of sick children rather than differences *between* sick and healthy children, is likely to be more fruitful in the future.

Single parent families

A further criticism that can be made of much work concerned with parenting healthy and sick children is that it is based on conventional two-parent families. It is well documented that the make-up of the modern family has changed dramatically in recent years. The assumption that a family consists of mum, dad and two children is being challenged from all directions. The modern family is one in which it is increasingly likely that the mother works outside the home for at least part of the time, with fathers taking more responsibility for domestic duties. Nevertheless, responsibility for everyday housework, shopping and caring for children, very much remains the prime responsibility of mothers, even where both parents work. Children traditionally remain with their mother when a family splits up, and given her reduced earning capacity, it is almost inevitable that some financial hardship follows.

The impact of chronic disease may be expected to add to the already considerable financial and emotional burdens of single parents. Financially, the additional costs involved in travelling to the hospital, arranging for other children to be cared for, and providing gifts or special foods for the sick child, may well extend the family budget beyond its limits. Emotionally, single parents may well be forced to shoulder the burden of knowledge relating to the child's disease and prognosis. They may have no single source of help in communicating with medical staff, and no-one to talk to about their concerns.

There is no established causal link between the presence of a child with chronic disease in the family and subsequent divorce. However, given the incidence of divorce in the general population, it is clear that many children with chronic disease are brought up in one-parent families. Despite this, little attempt has been made to consider the special problems confronting these families. For the purposes of statistical analyses, we may even *exclude* single parents from our samples.

As might be expected, single parents tend to report more stress than parents in intact families (De Maso *et al.* 1991). Limited resources can interact with additional care-taking demands to define some restrictions on the extent of the child's participation in everyday activities. Anderson *et al.* (1983), for example, reported that school attendance in children with asthma was comparable with healthy children except where they were being brought up in single parent families. Also in children with asthma, Christiaanse, Lavigne and Lerner (1989) found that adherence to treatment was worse in those from single parent families.

However, other work has not found such disadvantage to occur for all children in single parent families. Adolescents with diabetes from one-parent families were not necessarily in poorer metabolic control, nor less compliant with treatment, compared with adolescents from two-parent families (Hanson, Henggeler, Rodrigue, Burghen & Murphy 1988). These authors suggested that children in single-parent families can become more responsible and mature compared with adolescents in intact families. Similar conclusions have been reached from work examining responses of healthy children to the loss of a father (Kurdeck 1981).

Parenting practices and medical care

The research considered so far has focussed on the implications of chronic disease for everyday parenting; i.e. decisions about discipline practices or child independence, which are issues for all parents. There is a further dimension to parenting chronically sick children. This concerns the impact of parenting practices for the child's adjustment to the disease and attitudes toward medical staff and treatment protocols. In the next chapter, this question will be considered in more detail.

CHAPTER 8

Consequences of Parenting Styles for Children's Adjustment to Treatment

Stressors specific to caring for a sick child

Many of parents' worries are intangible and sometimes not very logical. They can worry that their child will have an accident, even knowing that the chances are quite slim. Told that the treatment is associated with 80 per cent survival, many parents work on the assumption that their child will be in the 20 per cent who do not do well. Other worries are more tangible and relate to specific practical problems that have to be overcome. In many chronic diseases, it is made clear to parents from the outset that they themselves are primarily responsible for their child's health. Thus, they must make sure the child takes prescribed medication, follows an appropriate diet, and keeps hospital appointments. In that many of these prescriptions do not make the child feel better and may interrupt other activities that the child would prefer to do, there can be some conflict between parent and child. Both may feel tempted to skimp on treatments, or put them off for the time being. Given the complexity of many treatments, the fact that they will not result in cure and often do not even make the child feel better, parents and children may question *why?* As a consequence, non-compliance rates in pediatric chronic disease can be higher than might be expected.

Compliance

Non-compliance rates in pediatric patients have been estimated to range from 20 to 80 per cent, and are comparable with non-compliance rates in adults (Litt & Cuskey 1980). Non-compliance rates in adolescents, however, are generally considered to be higher than among pediatric (Tebbi *et al.* 1986) or adult patients (Korsch, Fine & Negrette 1978). Among pediatric patients, non-compliance rates are almost wholly attributable to parental behaviour. However, during adolescence, patients themselves are encouraged to become responsible for as much of their own treatment as possible. Non-compliance can be attributed to adolescent's behaviour, parents' behaviour, or a failure to communicate responsibility between them.

Measurement of compliance

The terms *adherence* and *compliance* are sometimes used interchangeably in the literature. Compliance tends to assume more extreme, nonquestioning implementation of advice, *'the extent to which a person's behaviour coincides with medical advice'* (Haynes, Taylor & Sackett 1979). This definition implies a standard against which a person's behaviour can be assessed; i.e a prescribed regimen. The inadequacy of such a definition stems from the variability in advice which patients with the same condition may be offered; there is rarely a standard protocol. Given individual differences in the course of disease, it would be very inappropriate if such variability did not exist. Yet many investigations of compliance do compare patients' behaviour against a standard or ideal regimen, regardless of subtleties in prescribed information.

An alternative, increasingly acceptable approach is to measure the frequency of different health-related behaviours, without making comparisons to any standard. Such behaviours may subsequently be categorized as 'adherent' or 'nonadherent'. However, distinctions such as these tend to be arbitrary. The use of nonstandardised cut-off points restricts the possibility of comparisons across studies, or even across different aspects of the same regimen. (A population of children with diabetes may comply reasonably about dietary advice while essentially ignoring information about foot-care). Measurement of compliance is further complicated by the fact that it is far from clear what level of compliance is necessary for successful treatment. In order to overcome these problems, an alternative method is to concentrate on defining and measuring adherence behaviours, which has the advantage of placing adherence on a continuum, rather than subject to arbitrary cut-offs (for reviews see Cluss & Epstein 1985 and La Greca 1988.)

Family interaction and compliance in diabetes

Management of diabetes requires that children learn a complex and demanding set of behaviours and implement them at appropriate times. The extent to which they are successfully able to follow medical advice is dependent on many factors, but the attitudes and behaviour of family members can be quite crucial. Families can be supportive in helping the child deal with specific tasks, such as injections, either on a regular basis because the child is too young or inexperienced to perform the task alone, or on special occasions, such as when the child is feeling tired or unwell. Families can also be supportive by making changes in their own routines or diet in order to fit round the diabetes regimen. Despite good intentions, many families seem to be unable to offer consistent support of this kind beyond the initial diagnosis period. Families who enjoy an evening in front of the television eating crisps and chocolate can very much jeopardise the child's ability to adhere to recommended advice.

Even where families know what they should do to help the child, and are highly motivated to help, mistakes can be made, and relationships deteriorate. Parental efforts to help can be interpreted by the child as intrusive, and are seen as thwarting the child's efforts to manage the treatment and develop more autonomous behaviours. Analogous situations have been documented in other contexts. Coyne, Wortman and Lehman (1988) reported that the behaviour of wives of men recovering from myocardial infarction could often have the effect of jeopardising recovery by undermining the mens' efforts to do things for themselves. In essence, this process of 'miscarried helping' represents the negative side of social support; a failure of 'well-intentioned support attempts because they are excessive, untimely, or inappropriate' (Coyne *et al.* 1988, p.2.)

There is substantial evidence that poor family relationships, conflict, rigidity and lack of cohesion are all associated with poorer metabolic control in diabetes (Anderson *et al.* 1981; Bobrow, AvEuskin & Siller 1985; Shouval, Ber & Galatzer 1982). Although this association is well-documented, it is unfortunately not true that supportive family environments are necessarily associated with good control. Adequate metabolic control is dependent, at least in part, on physiological factors, including hormonal changes characteristic of adolescence, and residual insulin production, which are beyond individual or family control (Johnson 1988).

Nevertheless, there is some evidence for an association between family functioning, metabolic control and childrens' adjustment. Positive relationships between psychosocial adjustment and family functioning were reported by Grey, Genel and Tamborlane (1980). In a study by Baker *et al.* (1982), family supportiveness, competence and clear communication were associated with more adequate metabolic control one year later. In a further prospective study of 43 of these patients, Sargent *et al.* (1985) reported that positive family relationships were associated with haemoglobin control three years later.

The literature is confused, however, by studies which suggest no relationship between family functioning and metabolic control. Kovacs *et al.* (1989), for example, studied the relationship between family functioning and marital quality in relation to metabolic control in a cohort of newly-diagnosed patients between 8 and 13 years of age. Assessments of control were made on two occasions; at 3–4 months after diagnosis and again six years later, and included measures of glycosylated haemoglobin and weight-adjusted insulin dose. Family functioning was measured in two ways. Parents' perception of the overall quality of family life was measured by the Family Concept Inventory (van der Veen & Olson 1983). A sub-set of 48 of the original 80 items in this scale yield an index of Family Effectiveness. Areas of functioning such as openness of communication, ability to resolve conflict, family loyalty and satisfaction, and closeness of family relations were assessed. As a result of mothers' responses to items on this scale, families were categorised on a continuous scale, from poor to highly effective in family functioning.

There were no relationships between metabolic control or weight-adjusted insulin dose in relation to family or marital variables at either assessment times. Thus, Kovacs et al. (1989) concluded that it was not possible to predict metabolic control from the quality of family or marital relationships. Yet a small sub-sample of their population was characterised by both metabolic and family problems. Four of sixty (6.7%) were characterised both by poor family environment and inadequate metabolic control. Similarly, five of sixty (8.3%) of the children in families with marital problems, were later found to have poor metabolic control. The relationship between poor family functioning and less than adequate metabolic control may occur only in extreme cases of malfunctioning. For the majority of families, functioning at slightly inadequate or acceptable levels, there appears to be little evidence of a causal relationship.

It is also possible that inconsistencies in this area are attributable to methodological short-comings. Studies differ in specific instruments used to assess family functioning, with the result that different dimensions of family life are assessed from one research report to another. Many of these instruments rely exclusively on mothers' reports about family life, and therefore fail to account for the different perspectives undoubtedly held by fathers, siblings, or patients themselves. Instruments tend to assess global indices of family life, rather than specific dimensions which might be expected to relate directly to management behaviours.

Waller et al. (1986) found that good metabolic control was dependent on specific parental behaviours, in interaction with child characteristics such as age and gender. Good control was more likely where parents watched while the child tested blood-sugar levels, wrote down the responses and where someone in the family was available to talk to the child about diabetes. Boys were in better control in situations where families offered close guidance and firm discipline. Girls were in better control where families were warm and caring, with less emphasis on parental discipline. Aspects of parental behaviour associated with good control also varied with the child's age. Parental involvement in diabetes management (helping the child to implement procedures, reminding them about tasks to be done), was associated with good control in younger children, but relatively poor control in older children. It is very possible that this aspect of parent–child relationships contributes to the poor control which is characteristic of adolescents with diabetes. They may be resistant to much parental involvement in management and resent being reminded by parents about treatment requirements. At the same time, they may not have developed as fully consistent and reliable attitudes to their own self-care as necessary, (see Chapter 4).

The processes underlying the relationship between family functioning and diabetes management or metabolic control may operate either directly or indirectly (Hanson, Henggeler & Burghen 1987). A supportive family environment may effect health directly, by promoting good physical and mental health for all individual members. Alternatively, a supportive family may operate more indirectly, by creating an atmosphere in which it is relatively easy to adhere to treatment advice. Some support for this latter interpretation was provided by Hanson, Henggeler and Burghen (1987). Positive family relations (assessed by measures of marital satisfaction, family cohesion and adaptability) were related to good adherence behaviour, but not to metabolic control. This would be expected, given the relatively well-established finding that adherence and metabolic control are not simply related (Glasgow, McCaul & Schafer 1987).

Issues of discipline and control may be especially important in family management of diabetes. Families may experience some contradictions in their feelings about the child and treatment requirements. There may be some distress that the child has a chronic condition, which can be further aggravated in families with a history of diabetes. Parents of small children especially may feel sorry that they are not able to treat the child to an ice-cream or bar of chocolate, and at a loss about alternative 'treats' that might be offered. Dietary restrictions may create particular difficulties at birthday parties, and parents regret that their child is not able to enjoy these occasions as much as other children. Yet the temptation to treat the child has to be seen in the context of the implications of failing to adhere to the diet. Immediate fears that the child may experience a hyperglycemic attack as well as more long-term fears about future complications, may usually be sufficient deterrent. Parents may face numerous dilemmas as they attempt to balance the needs of the treatment regimen with a natural temptation to 'indulge' or more simply, treat the child. In some cases, anxiety about the consequences of non-adherence may lead to parents adopting overly rigid and restrictive approaches both toward diabetes related and more general child behaviours. The dilemmas may be particularly aggravated in adolescence, when the child's moves toward independence and autonomy may conflict with parents' concerns that the child does all that is possible to achieve optimum metabolic control.

Wertlieb, Hauser and Jacobson (1986) suggest that families of children with diabetes need to learn new rules about discipline and control; often adopting different rules about acceptable behaviour. In newly-diagnosed children, Wertlieb et al. (1986) found that behaviour problems were greater among children in families characterised by conflict. Fewer behaviour problems were noted in well-organised families, in which parents exerted adequate levels of discipline and control. These results were in contrast to comparable data for children being treated for acute illnesses. In this group, behaviour problems were associated with greater parental use of discipline and controlling strategies. The implication is that management of diabetes is best achieved within family environments where children are aware of, and accept, some measure of parental involvement and guide-lines about acceptable behaviour.

Some support for this assumption can be found in a study by Hagen et al. (1990). Although concerned primarily with intellectual functioning in children with diabetes, the authors also attempted to relate intellectual functioning to aspects of family interaction. Comparisons were made between families of children with diabetes and other families, based on the Moos Family Environment Scale (Moos 1974). Only one sub-scale distinguished between the groups; families with a child with diabetes appeared to be more highly organised. However, all the children had relatively good metabolic control (mean HbA1 = 10.7%), and therefore the sample may not be representative of a general population of children with diabetes. Nevertheless, it suggests that, in well-controlled families, the critical dimension of family functioning with any predictive value for metabolic control is organization.

At least with respect to adolescent patients, Hanson et al. (1989) suggest that the association between metabolic control and family relationships may be spurious. Correlations between metabolic control, marital satisfaction and family functioning were good under conditions of short duration of the disease. As duration lengthened, the correlations decreased substantially. Related analyses confirmed that the significance of the correlations decreased with duration of the disease, independently of the age of the child.

Non-compliance in children with diabetes is recognised to be relatively common, and perhaps reflects the fact that many people (children with diabetes and members of the public generally) do not see diabetes to be a very serious or threatening condition (Abroms & Kodera 1979). It is not a highly visible condition, not obviously life-threatening, and affects a relatively large proportion of the population. Individuals with adult-onset diabetes invariably have some residual insulin production, so that treatment generally involves attention to diet but does not necessarily include the need to inject insulin. The less threatening nature of adult-onset diabetes tends to colour perceptions of the childhood condition, resulting in a minimisation of the risks involved.

Family interaction and compliance in children with cancer

Although non-compliance is understandable in a condition which is perceived to be relatively non-threatening, it is less understandable in conditions which are more serious. It is often assumed that cancer patients automatically comply with treatment advice in order to maximise their chances of survival. Yet treatments are unpleasant and aggressive, often resulting in unpleasant side-effects and restrictions on everyday activities. The nature of treatment is such that children may feel very well before routine clinic appointments, but diagnostic procedures, anesthesia and side-effects of drugs have the effect of making the child feel sick, tired and irritable for some days afterwards. Under these circumstances, it is natural that children may sometimes question the value of treatment, and resist routine therapy. Patients may feel tempted to 'cheat' on treatment demands, or in extreme cases, opt out altogether, especially where they experience, or anticipate experiencing undesirable side-effects. At the same time, most treatment protocols are extremely complex and force patients into prolonged dependency on their parents. Non-adherence can result from a failure to understand the requirements of treatment, or disagreements between child and family about the reasons for treatment, consequences of non-compliance or issues of responsibility.

At a general level, non-adherence has been shown to relate adversely to the length and complexity of treatment (Haynes, Taylor & Sackett 1979); experience of side-effects (Smith et al. 1979); difficulty experienced in managing side-effects, and the degree to which the child's normal developmental functioning is compromised (Koocher 1986; Friedman & Litt 1986). Despite an assumption that children with cancer will comply with treatment advice, there is much evidence to the contrary (Smith et al. 1979; Dolgin & Katz 1988; Tebbi et al. 1986).

The relationship between the adolescent and family may be crucial at this time. Failure to communicate accurately about the change-over in responsibilities can in itself contribute to non-compliant behaviour (Tebbi & Koren 1983; Tebbi et al. 1986). Differences between adolescents and their parents in their perceptions of the relative importance of various aspects of self-care may further contribute to inaccurate communication (Levenson et al. 1983). These findings parallel those described by Anderson *et al.* (1991) that poorer compliance occurs where mothers and children with diabetes agree less about who is responsible for daily managements tasks.

Communication between families and children with cancer is, in any case, a particularly vexed issue, with many families preferring to 'protect' the child from such threatening information as far as possible. Chesler, Paris and Barbarin (1986) found that family characteristics, including sibling structure and religious beliefs, contributed to parents' decisions about how much information about cancer to share with the child.

Tebbi *et al.* (1988) studied compliance and parent–child agreement between 16 oncology patients, (aged between 9 and 19 years) and their parents. Compliance was assessed by (a) reports of having missed any medication in the previous month; (b) reports of how well medical instructions were followed; and (c) reports of the absolute number of missed doses during the previous month. Data were obtained separately from parents and their adolescents.

Non-compliance rates peaked at 47 per cent, at a point 20 weeks following diagnosis. The level of agreement between parents and their children differed considerably. A significant level of agreement was found on issues such as the required number of daily medications, frequency of medication and dose, and knowledge of how medication contributes to recovery. Agreement levels of approximately 60 per cent were found for responses regarding who was responsible for giving medication, knowledge of the correct time for taking medication, level of compliance necessary to effect a cure and level of satisfaction with information provided by health-care personnel. There was less parent–child agreement the younger the child.

There was some relationship between levels of parent–child agreement and children's self-reports of compliant behaviour. More compliant behaviour was associated with parent–child agreement on the following items; (a) agreed responsibility for administration of medication; (b) level of understanding of medication instructions; (c) ratings of medication effectiveness; and (d) knowledge of how medication effects a cure. Compliance in adolescents with cancer may be dependent on family relationships, and particularly on the effectiveness of family communication about treatment issues.

Family interaction and compliance in juvenile arthritis and asthma
Although there has been considerably less work concerned with compliance in conditions other than diabetes and cancer, the issue is still important. Evidence of substantial non-compliance exists for children with arthritis and asthma.

In asthma, Weinstein and Cuskey (1985) found that compliance rates were not predicted by child age, gender, race or duration of asthma. However patients on more simple regimes (three drugs per day) were more compliant than those on more complex regimes. Christiaanse, Lavigne and Lerner (1989) studied compliance in children with asthma in relation to family and patient characteristics. As reported by Weinstein and Cuskey (1985), patient gender and socioeconomic variables were unrelated to compliance behaviour. However, compliance was better among children from intact compared with single-parent homes. Children who were rated as better adjusted by their mothers were more compliant, but childrens' self-concept, self-competence and family organisation were not related to compliance.

In juvenile arthritis, it has generally been assumed that the family plays an important role in compliance (Fehrenbach & Peterson 1989).

Clinical manifestation of juvenile rheumatoid arthritis

Juvenile rheumatoid arthritis is a heterogeneous disease; different subtypes of the disease vary in clinical manifestation, disease course, and age of onset. The disease is characterised by unpredictable periods of exacerbation and remissions. Treatment is directed at minimizing inflammation and maximizing the degree to which the child is able to participate fully in physical and social activities. This is achieved primarily through physical therapy and pharmacological management. Patients typically receive an initial trial of aspirin, but more aggressive drugs may be prescribed as necessary. For the child, the real limitation is physical, but this can quickly have ramifications for social activities. These limitations, while presenting small children with difficulties, become more pronounced during adolescence.

Chaney and Peterson (1989) studied family functioning, knowledge of the disease and compliance in a small sample (n = 25)of children with arthritis. Compliance was measured in two ways. A global measure was derived, based on family member's estimates of typical compliance in relation to the prescribed dose. A second measure was based on a diary kept by the child and parent over a three-week period, in which they were to record medications as they were taken by the child. Overall, compliance appeared to be high. (Mean compliance score derived from the global measure was 96.0%, and from the diaries was 87.9%.) Even so, there were suggestions that compliance decreased with an increase in parents' perceived life stress; i.e. the more parents reported additional family stressors, the poorer was the child's compliance. Mothers' coping behaviour was particularly rated to compliance; where mothers had available a greater variety of coping behaviours, children's compliance correspondingly was better. Compliance was also related to fathers' satisfaction with family life; indicating that children's compliance with treatment is determined by the total set of relationships within the family, and not simply dependent on mothers' behaviour. Although it has been suggested that compliance is dependent on adequate knowledge (it is impossible to comply with a treatment regimen if you do not understand exactly what you are supposed to do), no relationship was found in this study between knowledge and compliance.

Difficulties in interpreting the compliance literature

For younger children with chronic disease, the family may be crucial in determining how well medical advice is followed and ultimately the success with which they are able to reconcile disease restrictions and treatment demands with everyday activities. Given the extent to which younger children are dependent on parents, it may be necessary to make some assessment of family functioning on diagnosis and throughout the course of the disease. Parents may need to be informed not only about details of the treatment regimen, but also how best to achieve their child's cooperation over time. It may be helpful if they are able to anticipate that many children can be difficult about taking medication, rather than experience this suddenly and without warning.

For older children and adolescents, the extent to which families are able to influence disease-related behaviour diminishes. Adolescence is, however, a particularly crucial time, in that power and responsibility needs to be handed over from parent to child. Confusions can arise through a failure to communicate accurately about who is responsible for specific tasks. Older children may be assertive in their demands for autonomy, but become daunted by the highly complex treatment requirements in many regimens.

Interventions to increase compliance behaviour need to address the concerns of both parents and patients, and work toward increasing agreement between them about the nature and implications of treatment and rationale for management protocols. This follows from findings such as those of Tebbi et al. (1988) that compliance is greater where parents and children agree about issues such as treatment rationale and differential responsibility. In many chronic conditions, there is an assumption that children should be encouraged as far as possible to accept personal responsibility for their own self-care, on the grounds that this will be associated with improved metabolic control in diabetes, and increased longevity and fewer side- effects in cancer. This view is increasingly challenged, as it is shown that children in the best physical control (who are presumably very vigilant about self-care) are also those in the poorest mental health (Close *et al.* 1986). The emotional investment required to achieve good physical control may create more psychological distress than is warranted.

The transfer of responsibility from parent to child parallels, and may often coincide with, transfer from pediatric to adult health care services, (see Chapter 4). Although it is to be hoped that these transitions can be achieved smoothly and without adverse repercussions for physical health, it is clear that there is considerable potential for confusion and disagreement. As is discussed more fully in Chapter 4, it is meaningless to consider any transition in isolation from the related physiological, environmental and family transitions that occur at the same time.

Parents' management of childrens' behaviour during medical procedures

Many parents wish to be with their children when they undergo medical treatment, and many hospitals encourage this. Children, too, often express a preference to be accompanied by their parents (Gonzales *et al.* (1989). Certainly for children undergoing brief hospitalizations for routine procedures, those who are accompanied by their parents experience significantly shorter stays than those who are admitted alone, (Taylor & O'Connor 1989). The results of this study imply that children who are accompanied by their parents recover more quickly than those who are alone, and are subsequently discharged earlier.

Yet it is far from clear that parental presence is beneficial for all children or under all circumstances. It has only rarely been demonstrated empirically that children benefit from parents' presence. Vernon, Foley and Schulman (1967) studied young children during anesthesia prior to surgery for tonsillectomies. Those who were accompanied by their mothers showed less distress than those who were alone. In contrast to these data, others have demonstrated that, at least on the surface, children can appear to be more distressed by their parents' presence during procedures than if they are unaccompanied. Shaw and Routh (1982) observed childrens' behaviour when receiving routine injections, and found that at both 18 months and 5 years of age, they cried more when accompanied by their parents. Gross *et al.* (1983) also reported that children cried more when accompanied by their mothers; this time when experiencing more painful venipuncture procedures.

In these studies, distress is measured in terms of childrens' immediate response to the treatment or procedures, and using these criteria, there appears to be some evidence that children cry more when accompanied by their parents (usually mothers). However, in these circumstances, mothers often have no real function to perform, and may themselves feel unsure about what to do and appear different towards medical staff. Children may use their crying to elicit comfort and reassurance from their mothers (Melamed 1992).

It is also possible that, having cried during procedures, children feel better and therefore, *in the longer term* are less distressed when accompanied by parents. Similarly, children who do not express their feelings during the procedure may feel more distressed for a longer time afterwards. Not all, but much of this work has involved pre-school children, and therefore it is not possible to ask them how they feel about their parents' being with them, or how exactly their presence is helpful or not. Whether or not children benefit from their parents' presence during medical treatment is likely to be determined by many factors, including the nature of the treatment, as well as characteristics of both parents and child, and the nature of the relationship between them.

Some evidence for the role of parents' characteristics (especially their own anxiety) as well as their attitudes to child-rearing has been documented in several studies (Bush *et al.* 1986; Dolgin and Katz 1988). It is hypothesised that mothers convey their own feelings and emotions to the child, (Escalona 1953), and by this process of 'emotional contagion' anxiety about the procedure is conveyed from mother to child. Research by Jay, Oxolins and Elliot (1983) supports this idea that more anxious mothers have children who are more distressed during procedures.

Bush *et al.* (1986) observed mothers and their children waiting in a routine pediatric clinic. Childrens' distress appeared to be dependent on characteristics of their mothers' behaviour. Children who were most distressed had mothers who were highly agitated, emotional, ignored the child and needed much reassurance from medical staff. In contrast, children who appeared to be less distressed by the proceedings had mothers who themselves coped well, and who employed a number of games and activities (for example, reading or playing) to distract their child during the waiting period.

Melamed and Bush (1986) suggest that the emotional contagion hypothesis may not completely account for parents' behaviour. Instead, they suggest that some parents may display such disorganised parenting when under stress that their children become excessively anxious, and this prevents the development of appropriate coping skills. Some support for this 'crisis parenting' hypothesis has been reported (Melamed 1992).

Although childrens' behaviour seems to be dependent on parents' behaviour during the procedure, it has not been easy to identify specific aspects of parenting which might contribute to the child's reactions.

Schecter *et al.* (1991) observed distress behaviour in 65 children, aged five years, receiving routine immunizations against diphtheria, tetanus and pertussis. One month before the appointment, children were visited at home, and parents completed a number of measures. These included:

1. Assessments of the childs' temperament.

2. Medically related attributes (is the child thought to be a good patient?).

3. Understanding of the purpose of pain and responsiveness when the child was believed to be in pain.

4. Predictions of distress at the approaching vaccination.

During the procedure, childrens' distress was evaluated by staff and separately by the children themselves. Generally, the children did not rate the procedures to be very painful; i.e. the average score was 2.57. (The scale used allowed for a maximum score of 11.) The children were subsequently divided into two groups; those reporting higher levels of experienced pain (2), and those reporting lower levels (≤ 1). There were some correlations between childrens' self-reports of pain and parents' ratings of childrens' temperament, so that those who reported more pain were more likely to be categorized as 'difficult' children by their parents. There were very few relations between childrens' pain or distress behaviour and parents' attitudes. However, parents' predictions about the degree of distress their children would experience correlated most highly with childrens' actual behaviour during the treatment. Schechter *et al.* argue that their data suggest considerable variability in childrens' self- reports of pain experience, while also demonstrating few characteristics of parent attitudes or behaviours which contribute to childrens' responses. These conclusions may be justified for relatively young children undergoing non-threatening procedures. However, parents' attitudes may become increasingly important with childrens' age, or where the procedures are perceived to be more critical or rated as more painful by the children.

While these initial studies focussed on children who were normally healthy but were attending clinics for routine or diagnostic tests, some more recent work had been concerned more directly with children who have a chronic condition. There is empirical evidence that behaviour in this context, especially the ability to cope well with pain and procedures, is influenced by parents' beliefs and behaviours. Dunn-Geier *et al.* (1986), using a videotaped parent–child interaction, showed that adolescents who did not cope well with pain had mothers who were more likely to discourage the adolescent's efforts to cope with an exercise task. Adolescents who coped well (no school absences in the last month) with chronic benign pain were compared with those who coped less well (missed at least three days school per month) in interaction with their mothers. Adolescents were videotaped taking part in a 15 minute exercise session. These exercises (sit-ups, step-ups) were chosen to simulate everyday activities in which the adolescents reported experiencing pain (for example, climbing stairs). Poorly coping adolescents and their mothers interacted differently together compared with good copers and their mothers. Poorly coping adolescents expressed more pain and were less often on-task compared with the good copers. At the same time, mothers of poor copers were more intrusive and tended to express more encouragement and discouragement – they gave conflicting advice.

Osborne, Hatcher & Richtsmeier (1989) reported that children with recurrent unexplained pain and their parents were more likely to report positive consequences of the pain and identify social models for pain behaviour in their immediate environment compared with children with explained pain and their parents. That is, those with unexplained pain had more relations with chronic conditions who supposedly acted as models about illness and illness behaviour compared with children with a known organic cause of their pain.

The need for regular and continual care can create many difficulties, particularly where treatments are painful and not obviously associated with improved health. The situation is particularly acute for some cancer patients, who are required to undergo many procedures, including painful venipunctures, bone- marrow aspirations (BMAs) and lumbar punctures (LPs). Some children develop such an aversion to these procedures that they become extremely anxious and nervous beforehand. Others develop 'anticipatory nausea'. In both cases, children's behaviour makes it very difficult to administer treatment, and staff and parents can become distressed by the children's behaviour.

Response to Bone-Marrow Aspirations

Dolgin and Katz (1988) studied parental behaviour in ten children with cancer who showed anticipatory nausea and vomiting prior to treatment, compared with parental behaviour in ten children who did not experience anticipatory nausea. Children themselves were assessed in terms of generalised coping and anxiety responses, using the State-Trait Inventory for Children (Spielberger 1973). Parents completed two additional questionnaires. The first was based on a *Child-development Questionnaire* (Zabin & Melamed 1980), and consisted of 14 hypothetical situations in which children might show fear or dependent behaviour, (such as going to the dentist). Parents were asked to select one of five strategies they might elect to use in order to manage the child. Each of the five strategies was thought to reflect a particular style of coping (positive reinforcement, modelling and reassurance, force, reinforcement of dependency or threat of punishment).

The results suggested some differences between children themselves in terms of who was likely to experience anticipatory nausea. There was a marginal tendency for those showing this behaviour to score slightly higher in terms of trait-anxiety. Perhaps more interestingly, there were also differences between parents. Those whose child experienced anticipatory nausea were more likely to report using threats of punishment and less likely to adopt strategies of reassurance than parents of children who coped with treatment without experiencing anticipatory nausea. A related study by Blount et al. (1989) demonstrated that some parent behaviours and vocalizations were associated with childrens' distress during BMAs and LPs. In particular, parental apologies or criticisms resulted in more overt distress behaviour by the children. Some parents became quite emotional, repeating 'I'm sorry' to the child throughout the procedures. Others were critical of the way the child responded; 'don't be silly; it doesn't hurt that much'.

These studies raise the question that childrens' behaviour in hospital may reflect aspects of parents' attitudes and behaviour, particularly their management of childrens' fear and anxiety. As observed by Rutter (1981), children may be affected as much by their parents' attitude and mental state as by any hospital procedures applied to them as individuals.

Dolgin et al. (1990) investigated this issue further, by comparing the strategies used by mothers to manage childrens' fear. Three groups were included: those with a child with a chronic life-threatening condition; a chronic non-life- threatening illness (including those with asthma and epilepsy), and a healthy group. As in the previous study, mothers completed a number of standardised questionnaires, including the Child Development Questionnaire (Zabin & Melamed 1980), the Hospital Fears Rating Scale (Melamed & Siegel 1975) and measures of anxiety. In addition, physicians were asked to rate the health status of the two illness groups, along four dimensions: illness course (stable, labile, deteriorating), prognosis (good, guarded, poor), degree of physical impairment (none, mild, moderate, severe) and visibility of physical residual (none, mild, moderate, severe).

There were no differences between mothers' reports of the strategies they would use to manage their children's behaviour as a function of the type of disease, or differences between the disease groups and the healthy children. However, mothers' use of threat of punishment decreased where severity and physical impairment were rated more highly by physicians. Mothers were also more likely to report using management of dependency as a strategy where childrens' health status was evaluated more negatively. Among children themselves, self-reported medical fears were related to severity and decreased with age. Mothers who were more anxious tended to use less efficient strategies to manage their children, relying more on force and threat of physical punishment and less on reinforcement and modelling.

These results suggest that management strategies were more dependent on childrens' health status than the specific condition. In particular, mothers of children in poorer health were less likely to report using threat of punishment as a strategy, and more likely to encourage dependency than mothers of children in better health, regardless of the specific condition.

Being with a child in pain or watching while the child experiences a painful treatment, is undoubtedly distressing for both staff and parents, and is clearly aggravated for parents who are themselves anxious about medical procedures. Unlike staff, parents have no clearly defined role to perform. Jacobsen *et al.* (1990) have described a typology of parent behaviours (see table 8.1). In their study, involving young cancer patients undergoing venipuncture, parents' behaviours and vocalisations, and particularly the *timing* of these vocalisations, were predictive of childrens' distress behaviour.

**Table 8.1. Operational definitions of parent behaviours,
(from Jacobsen *et al.* 1990)**

Parent behaviour	Operational definitions
Anxious questions	Says 'Are you afraid?' 'Did that hurt?' 'You look upset'
Bargain	Promises or offers future reward in return for cooperation, ('If you stop crying, I'll get you a toy').
Distract	Says 'Look at the drawing' 'Tell the nurse what you did in school'.
Emotional support	Hugs, holds hands, or gives other forms of physical or verbal comfort.
Explain	Says 'The nurse is going to take blood'
Plead	Says 'Please be a good girl', 'Please stay still'
Yell/threaten	Abrupt commands directed to child or future retribution, ('If you don't stop crying, you won't go home')

Overall stress levels were related to three variables: child age, venous access (a measure of the ease of accessibility of the child's veins) and parent expectations of cooperativeness. In line with other work, (Katz, Kellerman & Siegel 1980; Jay *et al.* 1983) younger children showed more distress than older children. Greater distress was also found in children with poorer venous access. As in the study described above (Schecter *et al.* 1991), greater distress was shown by children whose parents expected them to be uncooperative.

The two most common parent behaviours were trying to distract the child's attention and to explain the procedure and why it was being performed. Parents' use of distraction was not related to childrens' distress. The authors suggest that this is due to the fact that the venipuncture procedure is clearly visible to the child and therefore it is more difficult to distract the child's attention than during BMA or LP procedures (which are conducted behind the patient's back). The success of parent explanations in alleviating childrens' distress was dependent on the child's level of distress and phase of the procedure. Explanations were more successful when given at the out set to an already distressed child, suggesting that it is necessary that explanations are offered at a time when the patient is most likely to be receptive to the information. Parents' explanations aggravated childrens' distress when given inappropriately. In particular, distress increased where parents attempted explanations to already distressed children in the middle of procedures.

Parents' role in preparing children for hospitalization and surgery

There has been much debate about the relative merits of preparing children psychologically for hospitalisation and surgery. Previous reviewers have reached different conclusions about the success of psychological preparation, (Elkins & Roberts 1983; Eiser 1985; Goslin 1978; Peterson & Mori 1988; Saille, Burgmeier & Schmidt 1988). For the most part, research has focussed on comparisons of the efficacy of different methods, and characteristics of the child, including age (Ferguson 1979), or previous experience (Melamed & Siegel 1980; Melamed, Dearborn & Hermecz 1983) or issues relating to the timing of any intervention (Faust & Melamed 1984). Surprizingly little consideration has been given to the role of parents in helping to prepare the child, either before hospitalization, or during the intervention itself.

Yet there is some evidence that preparation of parents is important, and perhaps more important than preparation of the child alone. On the assumption that anxious parents make for anxious children, (van der Veer 1949), some interventions have been directed exclusively at parents (Skipper, Leonard & Rhymes 1968) or at both parent and child (Wolfer

& Wisintainer 1979; Pinto & Hollandsworth 1984). Other studies have trained parents, and then relied on parents to inform and train their children (Zastowny, Kirschenbaum & Meng 1986; Peterson & Shigetomi 1981).

As far as parental presence during preparation is concerned, results of most studies point to as much ambiguity as was described earlier, in terms of parental presence during procedures. Faust, Olson & Rodriguez (1991) compared arousal and heart rate in children undergoing elective ear surgery under one of three conditions. A control group was shown a standard preparation film including both procedural and sensory information (i.e. information about the surgical procedures to be experienced and the sensations usually aroused). In the other two conditions, patients viewed a slide tape showing a five-year-old girl modelling appropriate anxiety and relevant coping skills (for example, breathing deeply, imagining floating calmly on a cloud). Patients viewed the slide-tape either in the presence or absence of their mother.

Somewhat surprisingly, children who viewed the modelling slide-tape alone showed decreased heart-rate and sweating, compared with children in the other two groups. The results of this study suggest that the combination of a coping model and parent absence is associated with a reduction in arousal and anxiety prior to surgery. Provision of coping information may have led to increased self-efficacy among children, and, coupled with related observations that preschoolers tend to adopt dependent styles of responding to stress in the presence of their mothers (Reissland 1985) resulted in measurable reductions in physiological arousal.

The practice of utilising physiological measures of anxiety as indices of success of any program can in itself be questioned (Holden & Barlow 1986). There is little evidence for the reliability of these measures and alternative measures of childrens' distress or anxiety in medical contexts are needed. In addition it is important to recognise individual differences in desire for medical information. Some children thrive on being given as much information as possible about their disease and its treatment; others feel much more comfortable when they are not given extensive information.

Conclusions

Intuitively, we might expect a close relationship between children's response to treatment and parental attitudes. Parents can influence the child through a process of modelling; whereby through their own behaviour they provide the child with a clear message about appropriate ways of managing disease demands and restrictions. They can also encourage positive attitudes by creating a home environment in which communication about the disease and expression of emotion is allowed. Children need to feel that they can ask questions if they *want to*, as this creates an atmosphere of trust between parent and child. In some work in progress, we are finding that children with cancer seem to fare better psychologically where there is an atmosphere of open communication in the home compared with situations in which parents have been more secretive about the nature of the illness and reasons for hospital appointments. However, it often seems that what is important is that children feel some confidence that they can ask questions and will be given honest answers; in these situations they do not necessarily seem to have more questions, or be better informed about the disease and treatment than those from homes in which there is less open communication. Third, parents can encourage positive adjustment through establishing clear guide-lines within the family in terms of who is responsible for different aspects of treatment. A failure to agree within the family about differential responsibility seems to underlie much non-compliance, particularly during the late childhood/adolescent period.

There is some indication that poor parenting, in terms of lack of organisation, inconsistent discipline practices, and resistance to open communication, all contribute to poor functioning in the child and non-compliance with treatment. Unfortunately, there is far less consistent indication about what constitutes *good parenting* in the context of bringing up a child with chronic disease. Thus, within the literature on diabetes, it is clear that poor parenting is associated with fluctuations in metabolic control, but there are no indications that more consistent and quality parenting guarantee satisfactory control.

Research has so far failed to identify dimensions of sensitive parenting which make an impact on how children with chronic disease respond to the restrictions of their condition or rigours of treatment. The focus of much research is on parents themselves; how do parents manage the emotional consequences and how does this reflect directly on measures of parents' anxiety or depression? It is upsetting to see a child in pain, or have to accompany a child to surgery, knowing the seriousness of the situation. In these circumstances, it takes a lot of courage for parents to joke with their child, rather than reflect on their own anxieties. Yet where parents are able to turn the situation into a game, the child can draw considerable strength and gain confidence. Some parents can create a relaxed atmosphere for their child even in extreme circumstances. One mother told me how she achieved this. Realising that her child would have to spend a lot of time in hospital, and experience much pain and discomfort at the same time, she set about convincing her daughter that good things happened there too. They would make regular trips to the hospital hairdresser, even during periods when the child was at home. They also did their shopping at the hospital shop and would frequently visit 'friends' all over the hospital. From the beginning, the child associated going to the hospital with 'fun' and less with illness and treatment. Seeing this in writing, it seems obvious that these kind of activities would be helpful to the child. Yet few parents are successful; many prefer to keep hospital visits to a minimum and certainly would not make unnecessary trips.

The mother described above was lucky also; she had only one child. It was therefore possible for her to go out whenever she liked; she was also well enough off financially that she could go to a professional hairdresser often, and it did not matter if the prices at the hospital shop were a bit higher than in the main shopping precincts. Daily routines are much more complicated where there are other children in the family. School time-tables have to be adhered to, and the time available for play has to be shared out. Parents may express concern and anxiety about their sick child, but many harbour additional concerns about their other children as well. Healthy siblings can easily feel left out and almost jealous of the attention given to the sick child; parents face a tricky situation in balancing the needs of individual children. Everyday arguments between siblings are more complicated to handle where one child is seriously ill; decisions about how much to involve the healthy child or encourage a normal life are controversial. The impact of chronic childhood disease on other children in the family is the focus of the next chapter.

CHAPTER 9

The Impact of Chronic Disease on Sibling Relationships

Being left out

Having a chronically ill brother or sister is potentially one of the most stressful events experienced by healthy children (Coddington 1972). They face frequent separations from one or both parents as well as the sick child, disruption in daily routines and reduced opportunities to relax and interact with parents. Siblings can easily be overlooked by parents and medical staff. Medical staff may have little awareness of other children in the family, and their concern about social relationships within the family is more likely to focus on that between the parents (Bank & Kahn 1975). Healthy siblings have to work quite hard to attract parents' attention. One four-year old who had a baby sister with cystic fibrosis solved the problem by demanding physiotherapy twice a day for himself! It is perhaps not surprising that healthy siblings often seem to be the least adjusted of all family members, and most in need of support (Spinetta 1981).

It is inevitable, and natural that parents are preoccupied with the sick child, especially in the early stages of a disease. The stresses of this initial period can leave parents feeling drained, and lacking in any resources to deal with other family members. Their instinct, in terms of other children is often one of protection, and this can take the form of actively attempting to shield healthy siblings from any knowledge of the disease and its implications. This lack of direct information is frequently coupled with observable changes in family activities. Families can become socially isolated (Birenbaum 1970; Cairns *et al.* 1979; Crain, Sussman & Weill 1966; Kazak, Reber & Carter 1988); sometimes as a response to the perceived stigma associated with the condition, sometimes as an attempt to protect the child from general viruses and aggravated ill-health. Sometimes the isolation is forced on them, as other families feel impotent about how to help, embarrassed and uncomfortable about what to say, or occasionally panic that the disease is contagious. Eiser *et al.* (1991a) found that mothers tended to describe their pre-school children with asthma as very vulnerable; 'likely to catch anything that's going', and this attitude may well contribute to the limited social interactions and family isolation observed by others.

Common childhood infections, such as measles or chicken-pox, are potentially life-threatening for children with leukemia. Therefore, families must arrange that schools and neighbours tell them if any children have either of these complaints, and the child with leukemia be effectively isolated for the duration of the out-break. Where classes of children contract measles or chicken-pox one after another, it can happen that the child with leukemia misses school for a long time. Fear about how others will respond to the sick child, as well as realistic anxieties about contagious diseases, can result in families very much restricting their social lives. (This issue is discussed in more detail in Chapter 5.) Again, healthy siblings may be given little in the way of satisfactory explanation for this change in life-style.

Although parents hope for easy relationships between their children, the reality is often very different. Sibling interactions can be characterised by relatively harmless teasing and bickering, but they can also degenerate into more aggressive and distressing tensions. Yet for many of us, relationships between siblings are the most enduring of all (Antonucci 1976). Patterns of interaction established between siblings may well form the cornerstone of many other relationships throughout life. Children who have difficult sibling relationships tend to experience difficult peer relationships later (Dishion 1986). Poor sibling relationships in the preschool period have also been linked to behaviour problems and clinical disturbance four years later (Richman, Stevenson & Graham 1982). The assumption that patterns of interaction between siblings are important determinants of qualitative aspects of relationships with peers in later life is one reason why the study of sibling behaviour is currently receiving considerable attention.

Despite the friction that can colour sibling relationships, it is also clear that they can provide each other with mutual support and benefit. Older siblings serve a vital role in teaching and caring for younger children; in turn, younger siblings benefit from the experiences of older brothers and sisters, and generally learn from them. Good sibling relationships are especially important for children from disadvantaged homes, as they appear to buffer the impact of other life-stresses (Jenkins & Smith 1990).

Chronic disease threatens the integrity of the sibling relationship both directly and indirectly. Directly, opportunities for joint activities may be reduced and concern and anxiety dominate emotional ties. Indirectly, siblings may experience restricted activities and opportunities with parents whose energies are absorbed in management of the disease. In all families, differential treatment of children by their parents is related

to more conflict and negative behaviour between the siblings themselves (Boer 1990). Although research has often focussed on the negative
consequences which can follow the diagnosis of chronic disease, siblings
can instead provide each other with considerable help and support
throughout the crisis. Where there are several children in the family,
healthy siblings can exchange information between themselves. Older
children act as surrogate parents for little ones, easing the anxiety that
can otherwise be associated with parents' absence. Communication
between the sick child and healthy sibling is also important for both
children. It may be possible for either child to express doubts that they
feel would be less appropriately discussed with adults.

Nevertheless, following the diagnosis of chronic disease, many
healthy siblings are reported to show disturbances in behaviour, as well
as social and academic malfunctioning. For example, Carpenter and
Sahler (1991) reported that among 107 apparently well-adjusted siblings
of children with cancer, 61 (57%) subsequently showed signs of disturbed functioning. This included emotional lability (31%), negative
attention-seeking behaviour (25%), changes in academic performance
(22%) and withdrawal (16%). Other changes in behaviour, such as
somatic complaints, disturbed sleeping or eating patterns, and bed-
wetting or other regressive behaviours were also reported.

Parents themselves frequently identify concern about their healthy
children as an additional source of distress over and above that related
to the disease (Allan, Townley & Phelan 1974; McKeever 1981). Lack of
time to talk to the sibling is commonly reported. Parents may be busy
and fail to pick up on healthy sibling's difficulties. They then feel very
guilty that this only could happen because they were so wrapped up in
the sick child. Academic underachievement, and restricted play and
social opportunities are cited. Yet most of our understanding about
siblings' responses is based on *parents'* perceptions; do siblings' themselves see such problems and disadvantages? It would seem an obvious
question to ask.

While an obvious question, there are considerable methodological
difficulties. The first relates to gaining access to the children themselves.
Parents who encourage open communication and provide an opportunity in which adults and children can share their concerns rarely have
any reservations about giving consent for their children to take part. But
those who feel uncomfortable about involving healthy siblings, or feel
strongly that information will simply cause concern, may also refuse
permission for the children to be interviewed for research purposes. The
result is likely to be skewed samples. Second, a practical problem relates
to the fact that most research has included siblings across a huge
age-range, usually in order to achieve reasonable sample sizes. This

means, however, that developmental changes in siblings' perceptions of the situation, their emotional requirements and commitments to the family, and their available coping resources are undefined. Third, there are few standardised instruments available for the assessment of psychosocial and emotional functioning in siblings.

Siblings' understanding of the disease and their worries

Healthy siblings are often poorly informed about their brother or sister's illness. Motivated by a desire not to upset healthy siblings and a belief that they would be unable to understand anyway, parents often go to some lengths to protect these children from as much distressing information as possible. According to Burton (1975), 53 per cent of mothers of a child with cystic fibrosis had never discussed the condition with healthy siblings. When explanations were given, these were kept simplistic and minimal. In other studies, mothers reported that their healthy children rarely asked questions about the disease (Gogan, O'Malley & Foster 1977). Many mothers, who find it painful to discuss the disease, can interpret this to mean that the healthy child is unaware, or not interested to learn about the disease, and feel justified in not discussing the issue at all. Yet it seems that children may often be far more knowledgeable about the disease, and conscious of their parents' emotional response to it, than parents acknowledge. Children may fear that their parents are unable to discuss the implications of the disease with them and that their questions may precipitate a breakdown (Burton 1975). They can also sense a degree of parental disapproval associated with asking questions about the disease, and therefore prefer to keep whatever information they do have to themselves.

Few studies have systematically examined healthy siblings' knowledge of the disease or awareness of the prognosis and implications. Menke (1987) interviewed 72 children under 12 years of age with a sibling with cystic fibrosis, congenital heart disease, meningocele, or severe burns. Children were questioned about their knowledge of the sibling's condition, any related concerns or worries, perceived changes in the family and beliefs about how health care providers could help. Parents were also interviewed about their understanding of the siblings' awareness about the disease and their beliefs about the impact of the disease on the well child.

More than half the children expressed worries and concerns about their brother or sister. Worries largely centered on the prognosis, medication and the sick child's feelings. Healthy siblings also expressed concern about themselves and their parents. Many healthy children felt protective toward their sick sibling, and this was especially true of those who were older. Although 71 per cent of children reported that difficulties arose because of the extra attention that parents gave sick children, 59 per cent accepted the situation and claimed not to be resentful. Parents tended to underestimate the extent to which healthy siblings were worried about the sick child, and vastly underestimated, or appeared completely unaware of, concerns of the healthy sibling in relation to their own health and school progress. From these data, it is apparent that siblings experience a range of concerns and anxieties, which centre on the sick child, but include other more general aspects of their own lives. Discrepancies between sibling and parental reports suggest that parents may often be so preoccupied in caring for the sick child that they have no time or resources left to deal with the worries of other children in the family. Similar findings were reported by Walker (1988), again in relation to siblings of children with cancer.

A further study to describe the worries of healthy siblings was investigated by Harder and Bowditch (1982), this time in relation to siblings of children with cystic fibrosis. Their results point to the wide range of response that healthy siblings make toward the chronically sick child, and especially the degree to which experience of a chronic disease in the family can be conducive to the growth of empathy and consideration. Many of the siblings interviewed identified problems and concerns about the sick child, and described their own resentment about special attention that was directed toward the sick child. At the same time, the majority of the children appeared to understand the need for extra parental care and attention, and were resigned to the situation. This study is disappointing in failing to address concerns that might be expected specifically to affect siblings of children with cystic fibrosis. Given the inherited nature of the condition, siblings may be more likely to feel guilty that they are well, or be very conscious that it could equally be themselves who had the disease. At some time too, many have to face the fact that they are themselves carriers of the disease. The very demanding treatment may mean that siblings are forced into some involvement in implementing treatment. Responses toward peers who might tease the sick child is again an issue of central importance, but is not addressed in this study.

Psychological adjustment among healthy siblings

The difficulties that can arise for healthy siblings have been extensively reviewed in many previous articles (McKeever 1983; Drotar & Crawford 1985; Lobato, Faust & Spirito 1988). What is less frequently acknowledged is that other outcomes are possible. Some illness experience can enhance childrens' understanding of others, allowing them the opportunity to develop empathy and consideration (Parmelee 1986). More empirical evidence for this was reported by Horwitz & Kazak (1990).

These authors reported that preschool children with a brother or sister suffering from cancer were more considerate and helpful compared with age-matched controls who had no experience of the impact of illness on others. Other work suggests female siblings tend to choose careers in the helping professions, perhaps reflecting heightened awareness of others' suffering as well as a desire to be involved in help and care (Cleveland & Miller 1977).

Psychological follow-up of healthy siblings has tended to focus on measures of academic, school or social functioning. Most are limited in that they rely on parents' (almost always mothers' reports) about the child's behaviour. As such, they may be subject to bias reflecting mothers' anxieties about the sick child or misconceptions associated with disease-related depression (Lancaster, Prior & Adler 1989). Even teacher reports are not 'blind', and are invariably made with knowledge of the disease very much in mind. Very little attention has been paid to the way in which siblings themselves perceive their family relationships, or the impact of the disease on their lives. It is important that future work attempts to involve siblings more closely in research, since it is only by hearing their own stories that it will be possible to assess the short and long term consequences of chronic disease on their development. While their exclusion from much current work may largely reflect practical difficulties or ethical considerations involving the children in research, it creates a void in our understanding of sibling issues.

There are parallels between work concerned with adjustment in siblings of chronically sick children and that with the patients themselves. That is, although there are indications of maladjustment, especially from work which is conducted with relatively small samples of siblings drawn from specialist treatment centres, there is less indication of maladjustment from epidemiological work. Cadman, Boyle and Offord (1988) reported the results of a survey of 3294 children aged between 4 and 16 years – all had a sibling with chronic disease. Compared with the general population, there was a two-fold increase in emotional disorders, including depression, anxiety and obsessive-compulsive disorders. There was a 1.6 risk relating to poor peer relationships. Other conventional indicators of maladjustment, including conduct or somatization disorders, hyperactivity, school absence or low participation in leisure and recreation activities, did not differentiate siblings of children with chronic disease from the rest of the population.

This study suggests that overall levels of maladjustment are not grossly elevated among siblings. However, differences within the group which might identify child, family or disease characteristics which make some children particularly vulnerable, tend to be masked in epidemiological studies of this kind.

Results from other research, (which generally involve smaller, discrete populations) suggest that healthy siblings of chronically sick children tend to report more somatic complaints than peers from normal families. Sleep disturbances, eneuresis, appetite problems, head-aches, recurrent abdominal pain and a preoccupation with personal health have all been demonstrated (Lavigne & Ryan 1979; Kagen-Goodhart 1977; Peck 1979; Powazek et al. 1980). Miller et al. (1982) reported that siblings of young adults with rheumatic disease were at risk from self-perceived health problems, particularly asthma. Several hypotheses have been advanced as to why siblings show these somatic complaints. First, according to Social Learning theory (Bandura 1977), it is hypothesised that illness behaviour is learned from models in the child's environment. Where a child is frequently exposed to a family model who is ill, the child will learn this as an appropriate expression of behaviour, and will exhibit similar symptoms, whether or not these are appropriate. Walker and Greene (1991) showed that children with unexplained recurring pain came from families in which there were more relatives who had experienced serious illness compared with children with a known organic basis for their pain. Although not based directly on work with siblings, the implication may be that healthy siblings could be expected to develop more somatic complaints through a process of modelling the behaviour of the chronically sick child.

A second hypothesis is that healthy siblings may see that the way to gain parental attention is through the manifestation of physical symptoms. In this case, the somatic symptoms may be more parsimoniously construed as *attention-seeking* behaviour. Third, siblings may act out their concerns about the disease by developing somatic symptoms. They may be particularly sensitive to small changes in physical functioning, and more likely to express concern about the meaning of symptoms which others would regard as trivial. According to Miller (1987), individuals differ in the extent to which they 'monitor' symptoms (actively seek information), in contrast to those who 'blunt' (deny or avoid information; see Chapter 5 for a fuller discussion). The third hypothesis, therefore, suggests that healthy siblings may more often be described as 'monitors' compared with siblings from healthy families. To date, systematic work to address the processes underlying sibling adaptation to chronic disease in the family, is yet to be addressed. Scales specifically to assess monitoring and blunting in children have recently been developed (Lepore & Kliewer 1989) and are potentially useful in this context. In support of this third hypothesis, it has been noted that many healthy siblings do confess to being concerned that they too might 'catch' or have inherited the condition (Sourkes 1987), (although we have spoken to many siblings of chronically sick children who dismiss this as ridiculous).

Academic achievement and behaviour

Siblings are sometimes the focus of research work concerned with academic achievement or behavioural functioning, but are more often chosen as a comparison group when assessing the impact of chronic disease on the pediatric patient. In these cases, it is customary to include only those siblings nearest in age to the patient, since additional children cannot be considered as independent subjects. The logic behind this comparison is that it is assumed that there are considerable similarities between different children in the same family, given shared genetic and familial backgrounds. Any differences between the two groups are expected to be such that the healthy siblings will be superior at least with respect to academic functioning. Thus the implication is that any deficits in academic functioning in chronically sick children can be attributable to the disease process or its treatment, rather than social restrictions.

The assumption that healthy children will be relatively unaffected in academic achievement or behavioural functioning is necessarily naive. Healthy siblings are not at risk from side-effects of the treatment, but they may well experience difficulties resulting from alterations in parental behaviours and attitudes towards all the children. Concern about one child may lead to heightened concern about all children, or it may mean that parents are so overwhelmed and preoccupied by the sick child that they have little time or energy left for other children. Research work has focussed very narrowly on implications of chronic disease in terms of caretaking or domestic responsibilities of healthy siblings, with little account for the cognitive processes underlying parents' interactions with their other children. Neither has there been much attempt to understand the way in which healthy siblings perceive their parents or the consequences of their behaviour. Where there has been research, it has often been overly concerned with consequences for jealousy, hostility and aggression, with much less interest in healthy childrens' more altruistic concerns or anxieties about their own health.

School problems and maladaptive behaviours have been identified in siblings of cancer patients (Binger et al. 1969; Stehbens & Lascari 1974; Tritt & Esses 1988) as well as siblings of children with cystic fibrosis (Burton 1975), spina bifida (Tew & Lawrence 1973) and nephrotic disease (Vance et al. 1981). There are even occasional reports that healthy children achieve less well academically and are generally less well adjusted compared with their chronically sick siblings (Miller et al. 1982).

Social and emotional development

Until very recently, there was almost unanimous consensus that siblings of chronically sick children experienced adverse social and emotional consequences. There was an assumption that healthy siblings would experience jealousy and resentment because of parental concerns and attention paid to the sick child; guilt as a consequence of these feelings of resentment and jealousy; hostility; embarrassment over the consequences of the disease and fear arising from anxieties that the disease was contagious (Circerrelli 1982; Travis 1978; Tropauer, Franz & Dilgard 1970; Ward & Bower 1978). These observations were largely substantiated by later work using more structured and standardised assessment procedures.

In comparison with standardised norms, or in relation to matched control groups, a number of studies suggested that healthy siblings showed elevated levels of anxiety, fear and preoccupation with their own health. In addition, there was evidence of social isolation and hostility and aggression (Cairns *et al.* 1979; Lavigne & Ryan 1979; Breslau, Weitzman & Messenger 1981). Ferrari (1987) compared 30 children with a sibling with diabetes and 30 healthy children from families where all members were well and healthy. The groups were matched in terms of age, family size and socio-economic status. Siblings of children with diabetes were found to have lower self-concept scores and to have concerns about their own intellectual and school achievements, personal happiness and life satisfaction compared with children of healthy siblings. Harvey and Greenway (1984) reported lower self-concepts in children with a sibling with a physical handicap when both attended the same school, but not where they attended different schools. Perhaps the lowered self-esteem of the handicapped child rubs off on to the healthy sibling when they are in the same environment. As an indication of the extreme distress that can occur for healthy siblings, it has even been reported that they have lower self-concepts than their ill brother or sister (Carr-Gregg *et al.* 1985).

Other studies have not identified extensive adjustment problems in healthy siblings (Gayton *et al.* 1977; Lavigne *et al.* 1982). Hoare (1984) reported no problems among siblings of children newly diagnosed with epilepsy, although difficulties were noted among siblings of longer standing patients. In a separate study based on a different cohort of children with epilepsy, Hoare and Kerley (1991) found some evidence of siblings being affected, with 25 per cent rated as disturbed by teachers. These ratings were not confirmed by parents, which may in itself suggest that parents of sick children are more aware of, or ready to admit to, difficulties experienced by the sick child compared with healthy children in the family. These studies raise questions about the generality of adjustment difficulties among healthy siblings, suggesting that adverse effects are not inevitable, and that individual differences or family factors are important mediating variables. The lack of findings also raise more methodological questions about the adequacy of measures used to assess adjustment in the group. Although these authors did not specify adjustment measures, it is possible that the instruments used were insufficiently sensitive to uncover subtle deficiencies.

In contrast, there is a much less literature attesting to the growth of concern and empathy among healthy siblings. Iles (1974) described siblings of children with cancer as compassionate, tolerant, empathic toward their parents and appreciative of their own health. Both Grossman (1972) and Ferrari (1984) felt that healthy siblings were more sensitive and socially mature than peers who had no experience of chronic disease. Ferrari (1984) noted that teachers rated *younger* siblings of children with diabetes or developmental disorders as more socially competent than siblings of healthy children.

While few studies have examined the impact of chronic disease from a developmental perspective, there is an implication that it is younger siblings particularly who are likely to respond more altruistically. In a study specifically concerned with pre-school children, Horwitz and Kazak (1990) studied the implications of chronic childhood disease for the development of pro-social behaviour and sibling relationships. The study is exemplary in its attempt to elicit information directly from the siblings, rather than rely on parent reports.

Twenty-five children (aged between 3 and 5 years) took part in the study. All had a sibling being treated for childhood cancer. A control group of pre-school children with a sibling being treated for acute conditions was also included. Mothers completed measures of child behaviour (Achenbach & Edelbrock 1983), Family Adaptability and Cohesion (Olson, Bell & Portner 1982) and the Global Alike–Different and Sibling Attributes Scale (adapted from Schacter *et al.* 1976). These scales were included to assess parent perceptions of likeness or difference between siblings. The Global Alike-Difference Scale asks for a dichotomous judgment of likeness or difference. Mothers were also asked to rate their children on seven-point Likert scales, from 1 = 'very much alike' to 7 = 'very different'. The Sibling Attribute Scale consisted of 23 semantic differential scales (for example, neat–messy; withdrawn–outgoing). Mothers completed separate versions of this Scale for each child. Mothers also completed the Parents' Report of Prosocial behaviour, based on observation studies of prosocial behaviour in pre-school children reported by Dunn and Munn (1986). (Examples of items in this scale are 'comforts someone' and 'helps/pretends to help with chores'.)

Children completed two measures; The Pictorial Scale of Perceived Competence (Harter & Pike 1984) and the Different–Same game. The latter was a ten-item, illustrated game, in which children were shown pairs of pictures. Within each pair, there is a choice of two figures in the same or different pose, and children were asked to point to the pair most like them and their sibling. Total scores are the number of different pictures selected.

There were no differences between the sibling groups in adjustment, competence, nor in terms of their total scores on the measure of prosocial behaviour. However, siblings of oncology patients tended to have higher scores on five of the 14 items. These included helping, giving gifts, praising, sharing and showing affection. Thus, these children showed no evidence of maladjustment, and some evidence of enhanced prosocial behaviour. This may, of course, be as much attributable to the increased opportunities for prosocial behaviour which might occur in families with a sick child, and which would not necessarily be so frequent for siblings from healthy families. The presence of a sick child in the family may create opportunities for helping or giving gifts, which simply do not arise for children from the control families. While it is possible that children with healthy siblings would show comparable levels of prosocial behaviour under appropriate circumstances, the increased opportunities for such behaviour in families with sick children may ultimately be associated with more enduring differences between the groups.

Mothers of children with cancer rated their children as more alike than mothers of healthy children rated their children. In this way, they may be attempting to minimize the impact of the disease, by looking for similarities between their children.

A second study which again attempts to elicit information from siblings themselves was reported by Carpenter and Sahler (1991). Again, their focus was on siblings of cancer patients. Sibling's knowledge of cancer, and perceptions of the child with cancer were related to parents' reports about sibling adjustment. The Sibling Perception questionnaire was used to tap four dimensions of sibling behaviour:

- *interpersonal;* relating to interpersonal interactions and relationships: (I wish my parents would spend less time with my brother/sister; I don't want to bother my parents with my worries);

- *intrapersonal;* concerned with how the siblings perceived the disease to affect them; (I wonder why my brother/sister got sick; I feel sad about my brother/sister having cancer);

- *communication;* relating to parent- child communication:- (I can talk to my parents about cancer; I can talk to my parents about school-work) and

- *fear of disease;* (I worry that I can catch cancer from my brother/sister).

Siblings were divided on the basis of parent reports into those showing some problems in adjusting to the disease, and those who showed none. These two groups could be differentiated particularly with respect to *interpersonal* relationships, suggesting that siblings with adaptational problems perceived themselves to be ignored, unwanted and misunderstood, but also as not wanting to disturb parents with their own worries. They were more likely to perceive themselves as isolated (my parents ignore me); saw the illness as disrupting family life (we don't do so much as a family now); and lacked social support (I wish I knew someone who understands how I feel). The groups did not differ in their responses on the three remaining factor scales, nor in terms of their knowledge of cancer. Thus, children who were rated as better adjusted by their parents did not differ from those who were rated as less well adjusted in terms of their knowledge about the disease, perceptions of its implications, ability to communicate with others and share their feelings. Neither did they appear to be much more fearful about the consequences for their own health.

These results place less emphasis on cognitive or emotional response to cancer, but do suggest that adjustment is determined by family attitudes and behaviours, or at least, sibling's perceptions of, and beliefs about family dynamics and relationships. It is extraordinarily unlikely that parents deliberately exclude healthy siblings from the family, or consciously make themselves unavailable to listen to their childrens' problems. Rather, some parents may underestimate the impact of disease on healthy siblings, and need to be encouraged to relate more closely to them.

Parents and siblings may well also have quite different perspectives concerning the disease and its implications. Siblings tend to have less complete information and be less involved in decision making with medical staff. In addition, they may have specific concerns about the consequences of the disease for their own physical health, especially in the case of inherited conditions. Their previous relationship with the sick child is likely also to influence their perceptions of the situation.

A study by Craft and Craft (1989) suggested that parents and siblings do indeed differ in their perceptions about the impact of the disease and changes in family relationships. These differences were heightened among younger children. Siblings and parents separately completed a Perceived Change Scale (Craft 1985); a twelve item scale to ascertain perceived changes from the perspective of the healthy sibling. Changes investigated included; trouble sleeping, amount of food eaten, getting mad, trouble concentrating at school, getting nervous, fighting with kids, having night-mares, bed-wetting, nail-biting, wanting to be alone, wanting to be closer to parents, and feeling healthy. In addition to this structured questionnaire, siblings were asked to describe the most difficult situations they were required to deal with.

First of all, there were some issues about which parents and siblings did agree, mostly related to behavioural changes that occurred at home. There was much less agreement about changes in siblings' emotional responses, or experiences at school. Agreement between sibling and parent increased with the frequency with which the sibling was able to visit the sick child in hospital, but decreased with severity of the child's illness. Second, siblings were able to express a variety of concerns and fears about their brother's or sister's illness. Three categories of concerns were specially identified;- separation from siblings; worry about siblings and fear about the outcome of the illness.

There are few indications that healthy siblings show marked psycho-pathology in families where there is a chronically sick child. However, more recent work focussing on the emotional needs and concerns of healthy children suggest that many harbour real anxieties that are not recognised by their parents. Raising parental awareness about the emotional needs of other children in the family must be an integral part of any family-based therapy.

The need for bone-marrow transplants

Bone marrow transplants are currently used in the treatment of both acquired and inherited disorders. Among the acquired disorders are the leukemias, severe aplastic anemia and malignant tumors. Bone marrow transplants are only used for children with leukemia in certain circumstances. Children who are believed to have a poor prognosis with chemotherapy alone, or where primary therapy has been tried and failed, are the usual candidates. Among the inherited conditions are some immunodeficiency syndromes and metabolic disorders such as thalassemia or Hunter's syndrome.

Once this course of action has been decided upon, a suitable donor must be found. Only one child in four has an appropriate family donor. In other cases, donors are sought from the general public, or failing that, a partially matched family donor may be chosen, (although in these cases the chances of success are reduced). Preparation of the child for the transplant begins some weeks beforehand, and involves chemotherapy and total body irradiation.

The bone marrow itself is administered to the child through an intravenous line in a procedure similar to a red blood cell transfusion. To reduce the risk of infection, the child is cared for throughout in reverse isolation or a Laminar air flow unit. The child is not allowed to leave the room, but parents and staff can visit. Isolation lasts from 28 to 42 days (Barrett & Gordon Smith 1983).

Medical treatment is demanding and intrusive, with daily blood tests, administation of blood products and antibiotic treatments. Side-effects are common and extensive:

> 'Side-effects of the initial drug regimen are inevitable, such as the total loss of scalp hair, nausea, vomiting and mucositis of the mouth. Total body irradiation can cause lethargy and may have neurological effects in the long term... The child is restricted to the intake of freshly cooked, low bacterial or sterile food. When gastrointestinal disorders make oral calorie intake impossible, calories are given intravenously by total parenteral nutrition, which can lead to side-effects'. (Pot-Mees 1989 p.9.)

Psychological issues for donor siblings of bone-marrow transplant patients

As bone marrow transplants have become increasingly an option in the treatment of many childhood cancers, it has also been recognised as an extremely stressful option for all members of the family. The choice of a sibling as donor further exacerbates tensions within the family. Other siblings can easily feel excluded from the 'drama' of the disease, and strengthened in their belief that parents are neglecting them. At the same time, they express considerable ambivalence to the whole treatment process, and considerable relief that it is not necessary for them to undergo the pain and discomfort of surgery.

For the donor-sibling, a variety of emotions are generated. On the one hand, they have the opportunity to play a central role in the life or death of the sick child, and thus, at least for a period of time, become the focus of parental and medical attention. On the other hand, the donor sibling is confronted with the need for surgery and hospitalization and associated discomforts. Extended school absence is necessitated, creating problems academically and socially. Difficulties in school for the donor sibling parallel those experienced by chronically sick children themselves. Even beyond the initial treatment programme, donor siblings are required to be available to donate platelets or plasma for some time afterwards. (This procedure involves being attached to a machine for an hour or more at a time).

Given the investment of time and discomfort experienced by donor siblings, and the importance attached to the procedure by parents and medical staff, there is a real risk that donor siblings come to feel unrealistically responsible for the success or failure of the procedure (Gardner, August & Githens 1977). These authors also reported psychopathology, from mild to more severe, to occur in many donor siblings. Risks of psychopathology seem to increase where transplants involve twins or opposite sex siblings, and if the patient dies, or suffers serious complications (Wiley, Lindamood & Pfefferbaum-Levine 1984). There is a real need for age-appropriate information about procedures and implications of treatment to be made available for siblings of transplant patients (Wiley, Lindamood & Pfefferbaum-Levine 1984).

Bone-marrow transplantation is a relatively recent innovation, and therefore our understanding of the psychological impact on families, and particularly the dynamics of the sibling/donor-sibling relationship, is limited to the immediate or very short-term follow-up. The processes whereby siblings come to terms with events over a longer period, is far from understood. Both healthy siblings and donor siblings would appear to be very much threatened in these situations. They face all the disadvantages associated with having a chronically sick sibling, including parental absence and preoccupation with the sick child. In addition, despite the treatment, siblings may have to cope with the death of a brother or sister, complicated further by their own role (or lack of it) in the treatment procedures. Too often, support services are offered to the patient and parents, and the needs of healthy siblings are easily overlooked (Lenarsky & Feig 1983). There is a real need for age appropriate information about procedures and counselling both for donor and non-donor siblings (Wiley, Lindamood & Pfefferbaum-Levine 1984).

Effects of the death of a sibling

At least in the short-term, it is clear that the death of a sibling is a highly distressing event, and surviving siblings typically respond as might be expected. Guilt, anxiety, death phobia, disturbances in cognitive functioning, disturbed eating and sleeping patterns, separation anxiety, and distorted beliefs about death, the medical profession, hospitals and religion, have all been reported (Cain, Fast & Erickson 1964; Kaplan, Grobstein & Smith 1976).

Once again, family environment appears to be critical in determining sibling's immediate response to the death of a brother or sister, and the process of recovery (Bowlby 1969). Healthy siblings are dependent on parents for explanations about the disease and death, and are rarely in a position to benefit from social or emotional support outside the immediate family environment. They may be poorly informed about the death, and lack the cognitive ability to fully appreciate any information that is given to them. Adverse psychological responses among the surviving children are less in certain family situations than others. Davies (1988) studied siblings in 34 families who had all experienced the death of a child from cancer within a three year period. Siblings who showed better adjustment came from families which were more cohesive, placed greater emphasis on doing things together and expressed more religious or moral orientations to life. Siblings who appeared to be doing particularly badly came from families with few outside sources of support.

Siblings who were more involved in the impending death seemed better prepared and later report less disturbances in functioning compared with those who were kept at greater psychological and physical distance. Lauer *et al.* (1983) showed that siblings of children who died at home felt more positive about the experience than siblings of children who died in hospital. Those whose sibling died at home reported that they were more prepared for the death, received consistent support and information from their parents, and were involved in the care of the dying child. In contrast, those whose sibling died in hospital felt isolated, that their parents were unavailable as support for them and were unclear about the circumstances surrounding the death.

Although psychological outcome for the survivors may be improved if a child dies at home, it may be that some families lack resources to handle this situation. For these families especially, hospital care needs to involve the whole family, and professionals need to ensure that less visible members of the family are integrated in family decision-making and grieving as far as possible.

Variables that mediate sibling response

The presence of chronic childhood disease in a family undoubtedly represents a risk factor for healthy siblings. Yet maladaptation is far from inevitable. While some siblings do seem to be adversely affected, others show minimal maladaptation, and others apparently flourish. The wide variation in response suggests that many factors other than the disease interact to determine sibling behaviour. In reviewing much early literature, Drotar and Crawford (1985) concluded that there was no simple correlation between characteristics of the disease and sibling response; that maladjustment is selective and varies with age, gender and outcome measure; and that the impact of chronic disease is dependent on the dynamics of family relationships.

Age of the sibling is likely to be an important mediating variable. Younger children are less likely to be given information about the disease (Chesler, Paris & Barbarin 1986) and are less able to understand medical information (Potter & Roberts 1984). Their own development may be jeopardised because parents are preoccupied with the sick child. Parents often need help with additional care-taking tasks, including those related to the treatment of the sick child, and more routine care of younger healthy siblings. These additional demands can often only be met by older children in the family. Parents may be forced to rely on their older children for practical help, as well as using them as confidantes and sources of social support. Both Klein (1976) and Powell and Ogle (1985) have suggested that healthy siblings are frequently involved in more child-care and have greater responsibility for everyday chores compared with their peers.

Responsibility for domestic tasks may also be dependent on gender (McHale & Gamble 1987). Gath (1974) working with siblings of retarded children and Burton (1975) working with siblings of those with cystic fibrosis, all reported that the brunt of additional care was borne by sisters. Lobato, Faust & Spirito (1987) distinguished between brothers and sisters in the extent to which they were expected to be responsible around the home. Sisters of handicapped children had greater responsibility for child-care and domestic chores compared with brothers of handicapped children. In addition, sisters were given fewer priviledges by their parents and were more socially restricted compared with girls from homes in which there were no handicapped children. However, brothers experienced fewer restrictions and greater personal freedom compared with controls. The implication is that, although parents may rely on their daughters for practical help, they see it as inappropriate to use their sons in this same way. Perhaps also, girls are more prepared to see their roles in terms of helping around the house, and these differences between brothers and sisters reflect cultural stereotypes about appropriate behaviour, as much as bias in parents' expectations.

While age and gender of the sibling have received some attention, other individual characteristics such as intelligence, temperament, or beliefs about the disease can be hypothesized to be involved. To date, the role of these factors has not been systematically assessed.

Family demographic factors have also been implicated as mediators of sibling adjustment. In general, siblings seem to fare better in larger families, presumably because any adverse repercussions stemming from parents' involvement with the sick child are distributed across more children (Birenbaum 1970; Gath 1974). Perhaps also, the siblings derive some support from each other which effectively counters parents' pre-occupation. Impact as a function of ordinal position in the family is less easy to interpret, largely because age and ordinal position are inextricably linked. No clear pattern has emerged (McKeever 1983).

Psychiatric disorders among siblings of handicapped children vary directly in relation to social class (Gath 1974), raising the question that the impact of chronic disease may in fact be greater among middle, compared with working class families. Although chronic disease is one further disadvantage for poorer families, it is suggested that their lowered (or more realistic) expectations of life in general mean that they perceive the disease to add only marginally to their other problems. In contrast, for high achieving families, the impact of the disease may be perceived more negatively, as individual members see their ambitions and opportunities to be thwarted. In reality, the impact of chronic disease is currently understood only in relation to white, middle-class families, and this criticism can be applied specifically to work on siblings, as it can more generally. Directly and less directly, the way in which siblings respond is dependent on parental reactions, marital relationships and the family environment. Where either parent shows signs of severe depression or maladjustment, the healthy sibling may be required to take on an even greater share of responsibility about the house, as well as dealing with the emotional consequences of the parents' behaviour. Klein and Simmons (1979) compared chronically ill children with acute or serious renal problems, their healthy siblings and mothers. Evidence for the importance of family variables in determining sibling adjustment comes from the finding that healthy siblings had lower self-esteem in families where mothers perceived the renal condition to be more serious. Families in which there is open and honest communication about the disease would appear to create a more favourable environment in which all individuals can function, including healthy siblings.

Empirical support for this hypothesis is unfortunately limited, but the research conducted points consistently to the interdependence between sibling adjustment and that of the patient and other family members. Relationships between parents may indirectly affect siblings, partly by affecting the adjustment and behaviour of individual parents (Parke 1979) as well as their availability to the well child (Olson, Russell & Sprenkle 1983). Daniels et al. (1986) reported a study involving 72 children with rheumatic disease and 60 siblings of healthy children. The incidence of psychosomatic, behavioural, emotional and social problems was based on interviews with both parents and siblings. Those with a sibling with rheumatic disease reported a higher incidence of allergies and asthma compared with siblings in healthy families. Interpretation of this finding is complicated, however, since it may be attributable to a shared IgA deficiency in families with a child with rheumatic disease. Children with a chronically sick sibling actually reported more self-confidence, more involvement in family and other activities and better social integration in school than siblings from the healthy families. These findings contrast with other work and clinical assumptions that siblings of sick children are likely to lead restricted lives, with limited opportunities for play and interaction outside the family.

However, variability in sibling adjustment was considerable, although not related to the severity of the sick child's condition or extent of physical disability. Instead, adjustment of both the patient and mother, and family cohesion and expressiveness, were predictive of sibling functioning.

Implications of chronic disease for sibling relationships

Chronic disease affects the development of both the ill child and healthy siblings (Feeman & Hagen 1990). The authors report that the disease can create a shift in family heirarchies so that the sick child is treated as younger, and healthy children as older, whatever their ordinal positions. Chronic disease has a direct effect on all children in the family through changes in personality and self-concept, and an indirect effect through the changes that occur in parenting and parent–child relationships.

Although it has been argued that a systemic approach to understanding the impact of chronic disease on the family is necessary, most of the work reviewed has been restricted to an analysis of the perceptions of individual siblings and an assessment of their beliefs about the disease and its impact on their lives. The question of how the disease modifies sibling relationships and interactions together has received less attention. Evidence that qualitative aspects of interactions between siblings makes an independent contribution to the health of the sick child, over and above that of parent–child relationships, is provided in a study by Hanson et al. (1992). The extent to which adolescents with diabetes appeared to accept the disease and show appropriate, non-acting out behaviours was inversely related to the degree of sibling conflict. The authors suggest that '... parent-child dyads and sibling dyads represent interrelated and independent subsystems within the family, and that both subsystems may influence the psychosocial functioning of youths with IDDM' (Hanson et al. 1992, p.104). The role of healthy siblings in promoting positive adjustment and appropriate self-care in the chronically sick child may be a potentially fruitful area of intervention, but one which is so far unexplored.

Developmental changes in siblings' relationships

Work concerned with siblings' responses and adjustment to chronic childhood disease has paralleled but lagged considerably behind work with the patients themselves. There has been much similarity in the questions asked, empirical methods adopted, and theoretical paradigms which dominate the literature in both areas. The relatively restricted work on siblings, however, leaves many questions unanswered. In particular, there are considerable inconsistencies in research findings which make it difficult to determine the effects of characteristics of siblings, families or disease which render individuals more or less resistant to adverse repercussions.

Although there has been some attempt to describe the impact of disease as a function of sibling age, this has frequently been restricted to questions of responsibility for domestic routines and care of the sick child. Yet even this narrow focus has failed to achieve consensus; it is apparent that responsibility is dependent on a number of variables including sibling age and gender, family functioning, birth order, spacing between children and specifics of the disease. There has been virtually no research concerned with issues such as understanding of the disease, or concerns and anxieties from a developmental perspective. The same criticism can be leveled at issues of general sibling adjustment, behaviour and achievement in school, or perhaps of greatest significance, questions relating to the siblings' interaction and relationship with each other.

In common with many other themes identified in this book, research has traditionally been conducted from a pathological perspective; i.e. with an emphasis on difficulties, failures and deviance from 'normal'. Thus, our understanding of siblings' psychological responses is very much flavoured by investigations of concepts such as hostility, aggression, resentment and jealousy. Innovations in research which emphasise the impact of chronic disease on prosocial and empathic behaviour are certainly welcome, as too, are studies which consider sibling interaction from more developmental perspectives (Dunn 1987; 1988).

There are some lessons to be learned from research concerned with siblings of physically and mentally handicapped children. Some of this gives greater insight into family dynamics from a more behavioural perspective than is frequently employed in studies of chronically sick children. A greater variety of methods have also been reported, including telephone interviews and home-based observations (McHale & Gamble 1988). One conclusion from this latter study was that conflict between disabled and healthy sibling was not greater than that between normal siblings, but was perceived to be more problematic by the healthy sibling. A critical determinant of adjustment was the kind of attributions made by the healthy child about the sibling's behaviour. The role of attributions, particularly the extent to which disabled or sick children are seen to be responsible for their own actions and behaviours must take a more central role in future work. Developmental changes in attributions and the consequences for sibling adjustment and interactions, must be a fruitful area for study. Given changes in the make-up of the contemporary family, future work also needs to consider other categories of siblings, including step- or half-siblings (Treffers *et al*. 1990).

In many cases, healthy siblings feel excluded from family life following diagnosis of a chronic disease in another child. This can occur because parents genuinely believe that they are protecting healthy siblings from anxiety. In their efforts to ensure that life for other children is not affected, they can create a situation in which it is difficult for healthy siblings to find out about the disease. As a consequence, healthy siblings come to perceive a special relationship between parents and the sick child. This in turn can be interpreted as a rift between the healthy siblings and their parents. The existence of a special relationship can be reinforced by medical staff, who rarely think to involve healthy siblings in hospital routines; far less have time to give satisfactory explanations. Yet there are indications that healthy siblings would very much appreciate greater involvement. Stewart *et al*. (1992) interviewed 10 healthy siblings, each with a brother or sister with a terminal illness. None of the children had ever discussed the illness with a doctor, although three of the older children would like to do so. Although work with siblings lacks a clear theoretical framework, and suffers from many methodological short-comings, it does indicate that there is room for many practical improvements in management of these children. Some group-work has been reported and is to be encouraged. Pediatricians also need to acknowledge that they have some obligations to healthy siblings, especially in answering questions about medical issues. In being prepared to talk to siblings, pediatricians also signal to the children that they are not excluded from the hospital and decisions which are made there.

Choice of abnormal psychology as a yardstick has resulted in a number of anomalies and inconsistencies. For example, within a normal developmental framework, it is assumed to be desirable that children are involved in and responsible for some domestic and house-keeping chores (McHale *et al*. 1990). Yet much work concerned with sibling responsibilities in families with a sick or disabled child seems to make the assumption that such involvement is damaging and unnatural. Again, there is an assumption that differences in the way in which parents manage sick and healthy siblings are entirely attributable to the disease or handicap. Yet most adolescents believe that they experienced different family environments, and further parents themselves perceive differences in their treatment of children in the same family (Daniels *et al*. 1985). Failure to conduct research against a background which takes into account normal family relationships and sibling development very much restricts interpretation of the literature to date.

CHAPTER 10

Towards a Comprehensive System of Care for Children with Chronic Disease

'Psychological and support services are a central component of the ongoing care of children with chronic physical conditions (Brewer *et al.* 1989). It is no longer considered sufficient to provide biomedical care and technologically sophisticated interventions without appropriate attention to the psychological and social impact of both the child's condition and treatment' (Sabbeth & Stein 1990).

While many would be happy to endorse this point of view, practical provision of psychosocial care for chronically sick children remains patchy and often poorly integrated with medical services. Advice to mothers is generally poor (Stein, Jessop & Reissman 1983), and children themselves rarely receive the psychological help and support they need. This lack of care can partly be attributable to the fact that children receive care in a variety of different settings and typically need a range of services throughout their treatment. A child with cancer, for example, may initially be referred from the family doctor to a local hospital. Here tests may be carried out and the child referred to a regional hospital specialising in the care of children with cancer. Children may be referred yet again if they need specialist surgical or neurological treatment. Later, children may be required to attend all three hospitals for check-ups; the local hospital may conduct frequent, routine checks, the regional centre may wish to check for indications of development of secondary cancers, and the specialist surgical unit will recall the child to check on the healing of scar tissue. If the child develops an ordinary cold, parents feel confused about where to go for advice. The family doctor may refuse to see the child, especially if there was some confusion or indicators of poor judgment in the original decision or speed of diagnosis. The local hospital also has reservations about seeing the child, feeling that this problem is not related to the cancer and should be dealt with in the community. The result is that the family feels dissatisfied about the relationship between services, and anxious about how to gain the best type of care for their child.

In addition to health problems related to the illness, children also experience general health difficulties similar to their peers. Anxiety, drug and alcohol related problems, headaches, acne and dental problems have all been reported, especially among adolescents. Specialists in the care of chronic disease may be reluctant, or feel inexperienced, as to how to deal with these problems. However, since the specialists are acknowledged to be the key carers for these children, local physicians may be uninvolved and unaware of the needs of children with chronic disease. Carroll *et al.* (1983) found that 44% of a sample of chronically ill adolescents received no advice or care regarding general health needs, but relied instead on the primary physician. Only 27% of the sample spoke to the physician about their problem, reflecting perhaps a common belief that such people are too busy to be bothered with what are perceived to be minor or trivial problems.

Barriers to good psychosocial care also stem from the attitudes of the families, specialist medical teams and the psychological service providers themselves (Sabbeth & Stein 1990). The families may resent suggestions that they are not coping well and therefore feel reluctant to recognise their need, or accept additional help. In addition, families who are already burdened by appointment demands for medical care may feel unable to commit themselves to extra trips to the hospital. They also have reservations about the effects on healthy siblings, who may frequently be left in the care of others in order for the family to keep medical appointments. The potential merits of psychosocial care for the sick child need to be balanced against the disadvantages to the healthy siblings of interrupted routines and multiple caretakers.

Medical staff often have considerable confidence in their own abilities to manage psychosocial care for their patients, and feel reluctant to refer them to other services. Limited experience with children in the general population can mean that they are unsure about the variability in normal development, and medical staff may therefore dismiss as illness related problems that would warrant specialist help in children without chronic disease. The tendency to refer for psychological help only those children in extreme circumstances means that many failures are experienced in medical-psychological liaison. The result is that medical staff often express considerable reservations about the efficacy of psychological interventions.

Psychosocial staff, too, may be unwilling to accept children with chronic diseases as part of their routine case-load. Again, lack of training and medical knowledge contribute to feelings of inadequacy and uncertainty about how to deal with these children. Ambiguities in the relationship between medical care-giver and psychologist add to a reticence to become involved with chronically sick children and their families.

'Opinions differ about how much a therapist should know about the child's particular disease and its treatment in order to deal effectively with the mental health issues. Some therapists who work with many children with one particular disease, think they are ill-equipped to work with children with other disorders. They consider it essential to learn about coping with each particular disorder and its treatment. Others take a more generic approach, and believe that they can work effectively with the mental health issues without much experience with the individual physical condition' (Sabbeth & Stein 1990, p.76).

Theoretical issues

The value of a non-categorical approach

According to some workers (Stein & Jessop 1984; Varni & Wallander 1988), there are many more similarities than differences between chronic conditions in terms of the impact on child and family. Thus, the particular diagnosis is less critical than the practical, emotional or financial restrictions that are common to all diseases. In many ways, this is a potentially more parsimonious explanation than one which holds that all diseases have unique limitations and need discrete interventions. The implications of the non-categorical approach are that all children with chronic diseases face certain restrictions and disadvantages. Therefore interventions require related and integrated approaches, regardless of the specific disease.

In the work reviewed in this book, it is clear that it is not possible to distinguish between these approaches. Certain conditions, notably cancer, diabetes, and to a lesser extent spina bifida or cystic fibrosis, account for the vast majority of published research. Asthma, though by far the most common chronic condition of childhood, has received much less attention than more rare conditions. Other diseases, admittedly rare, such as renal disease, have received sporadic attention. Still other conditions, such as epidermolysis bullosa (a hereditary dermatological disease) have received virtually no attention at all (cf. Lansdown et al. 1986). Furthermore, most research is non-comparative and limited to considering the consequences of one condition. More extensive work involving more than one disease group is called for and will require collaboration across specialist centres.

However, the practical difficulties in establishing such a research program should not be under-estimated. Diseases differ along a number of dimensions (see Chapter 1). Careful recruitment of patients would be required to control for the effects of severity, extent of restrictions or amount of self-care involved when comparing different conditions. Very few studies to date have been designed explicitly to compare the non-categorical with alternative approaches to understanding the impact of chronic disease.

In all probability, both extreme positions are likely to be inadequate. There are certainly many difficulties that are shared by children with chronic disease and their families, regardless of the specifics of the condition. Hospital appointments, communicating with doctors, managing painful treatment, explaining the restrictions and implications to friends, all come into this category. In terms of practical provision of resources, there are circumstances when it is advantageous to consider children with a chronic disease from a non-categorical perspective. Hospitals need policies in relation to hospital–school liaison, in relation to education of children about their disease, in relation to involving siblings in disease management, whatever the specific label attached to the child's condition.

Measurement issues
The development of appropriate measures
In the drive for statistical acceptability, we have come to rely on a finite number of instruments, which may be defensible from the perspective of experimental psychology, but have little face validity. Good internal reliability can easily be achieved by including a number of items in questionnaires which, with minor changes in wording, essentially ask the same thing. For example, the self esteem scale to be completed by teachers (Harter 1985) is a widely used and statistically sound instrument. Yet there is much overlap in the items asked (the child's self-esteem in relation to physical appearance, for example, is assessed from the following items: this child is good-looking; this child has a nice physical appearance; this child isn't very good-looking). British teachers do not take well to being asked this kind of information about a child. Many questionnaires, which are reported to have good test-retest reliability, achieve this by including too many similar items, and are consequently too long, especially for use with sick children or harassed parents. Problems identified by Holden and Edwards (1989) in the construction of questionnaires to assess parenting behaviour, can all equally be applied to many instruments commonly used to assess the impact of chronic disease on children and their families (see Chapter 8).

There is a problem, too, in the kind of issues that have received most attention from research psychologists and psychiatrists; a consistent orientation to assessing adjustment/maladjustment and describing predictors of adjustment. Although this orientation was initially criticised some years ago, it is still very prevalent in much research.

'There is a regrettable tendency to focus gloomily on the ills of mankind – It is unusual to consider the factors that promote support, protect and ameliorate problems' (Rutter 1979, p.49).

The problem in all this work is that we have used normal families as standards against which to assess adjustment, tests developed for normal populations as our measures, and failed to get to grips with the uniqueness of the experiences of the chronically sick child. In hanging on to our standardised tests, we have gained little insight into the processes underlying adjustment or maladjustment. Only by considering more carefully the processes, or causes underlying adjustment problems, can appropriate interventions be adopted.

Theory and practice

Despite the increasing amount of research concerned with psychosocial issues in chronic conditions, very little can be said to have an impact on practice. Yet this must surely be the criterion against which success is to be judged. To achieve significance at an applied level, research needs to be guided by both pediatrics and psychology. Where questions are defined by pediatricians alone, they may focus on medical issues, and assign psychological issues a secondary role. Where questions are defined by psychologists alone, they can be theoretically derived and more acceptable (to academic psychologists), but lack obvious relationships to practical concerns. Much psychological work is unacceptable to the medical profession because it is too distant from what is perceived to be the real question.

'Clinical research in behavioural pediatrics cannot be a spectator sport but is best done by those who are actively caring for children with problem behaviours' (Haggerty 1988, p.179).

Real practical issues, which could best be served by joint approaches is only recently and occasionally coming under scrutiny. Examples include assessments of how to give distressed parents information about the disease at diagnosis, or how to gain truly informed consent to treatment (Lesko *et al.* 1989).

Barriers to effective medical psychological collaboration

As discussed above (Sabbeth & Stein 1990), barriers to medical psychological collaboration can be put up by families, medical and psychosocial staff. However, even where a referral is made, problems can be encountered resulting from unrealistic expectations from all parties as to what can be achieved and how those involved can best work together. Staff are often unclear about what other professionals can offer, and ignorant about their styles of working. The prevailing model of psychological care is at the level of psychologist/individual patient, with little evidence of collaboration between professionals. This has been described as the 'independent-functions model' (Roberts 1986), or noncollaborative approach (Drotar 1978). The psychologist is generally referred a patient by the pediatrician, makes an independent assessment of the problem, and refers a report back to the medical staff. The patient may then be referred elsewhere for follow-up or intervention, as a result of decisions taken unilaterally by medical staff.

An alternative model, again described by Roberts (1986), is the 'indirect psychological consultation model'. As in the previous model, the pediatrician retains responsibility for the child and family, but the psychologist offers advice and suggestions about suitable courses of action. Again, this process involves no real collaboration between different professionals.

A third model, the 'collaborative-team model' occurs where various professionals work together to provide a comprehensive service for children and their families. These approaches characterise specialist care, usually in large centres and invariably involving children with life-threatening conditions. Thus, centres specialising in the care of children with cancer may work through a health-care team. Medical staff have the responsibility for implementing the child's medical treatment, but in addition a social worker may help the family to obtain financial and other resources and put individual families in touch with each other. Pediatric nurses are specially responsible for preparing the child for procedures and providing medical assistance. They also make home-visits to help parents cope with some treatments at home, thereby reducing length of hospital stay. The psychologist may be involved in pain- management, liaise with schools, help children understand and come to terms with the treatment, and generally encourage other staff to be aware of developmental issues involved. All staff may share responsibility for helping parents understand the reasons for medical treatments, and provide support and counselling to families of patients on treatment, as well as keeping in touch with the bereaved.

Although this model is most common in centres specialising in the care of children with life-threatening conditions, it has also been adopted in centres specialising in the care of children with diabetes. Although it is not life-threatening, diabetes involves so much self-care that non-medical support staff serve an important function in education and encouragement for these children and their families.

Two facts point to the value of the team approaches described above. The first is that survival of children with cancer is better where they are treated in specialist centres involving collaborative care (Stillar et al. 1989). The second is that haemoglobin control is better in children with diabetes cared for in specialist centres than with those treated in non-specialist units (Bloomfield & Farquhar 1990).

Even in centres with established multi-disciplinary teams, confusions can occur between professionals, as to individual areas of expertise. Differences in background and training mean that other professionals are often not immediately aware of the contributions that a psychologist can make to comprehensive care. Indeed, communicating with other professionals, is frequently identified as a source of stress, especially by nursing staff (Cull 1991). In addition, medical staff have some confidence in their own abilities to handle psychological problems (Olson *et al.* 1988).

The role of the psychologist

The role of the psychologist has traditionally been seen in terms of intervention during crises. Too often, too little help is requested, too late. While it is becoming more common that a psychologist is attached to a specialist unit dealing with life-threatening conditions, it is rare that children with chronic diseases and their families are offered routine, non- crisis orientated psychological help. This situation needs to be changed for two reasons.

The first reason relates to the fact that by intervening earlier in the crisis, escalation of the problem into a major event can hopefully be reduced. Routine availability of psychological help should be associated with earlier presentation of problems, and greater manageability.

Second, the children themselves may encounter problems which are not specifically disease-related. These problems may be normal and experienced by all children of a similar age. Decisions about examination choices to be made at school, or interpersonal problems encountered in relationships with other children in the class, come into this category. Other problems may be family-related; arguments with siblings, for example, or anxieties about parents' health or relationships with each other.

Some of these issues may seem trivial, especially to an outsider, and in comparison to the potential problems associated with the disease. In addition, they may be played down by the child and family, as well as medical staff, precisely because they parallel problems faced by healthy children of similar age. Even trivial problems can seem large to the individual, and can take on more gigantic proportions where other life-stressors, such as disease and treatment are already part of the daily stress load. The very fact that the children are under hospital care can further reduce their access to non-medical support and help. Children who have supposedly been 'cured' of cancer very much come into this category. Although hospital staff are keen to check them at specified intervals, they tend to trivialize what appear to be minor aches and pains, on the grounds that these reflect unnecessary anxiety rather than genuine illness. Local doctors are also reticent about treating the children, in that they do not consider themselves to be experts in caring for children with cancer, even if it is cured. The result is that the child feels there is nowhere to go, and receives less adequate care than any other child in the general population.

Generally referred problems

What kind of issues generally come to the attention of psychologists working with chronically ill children? In one of the earliest surveys relevant to this issue, Drotar (1978) found that over half the referrals to psychologists working in hospital settings were for developmental or intellectual problems associated with physical illness, language disabilities or deprivation. Referrals concerning the management of chronic disease, adjustment to burns, child abuse and accidents accounted for another 30 per cent. Less than 10 per cent of referrals were for behavioural or psychiatric problems. A more recent report by Olson *et al.* (1988) found that 42 per cent of the work-load was accounted for by children with medically related problems. The most frequent referrals were for depression or suicide attempts, poor adjustment to the illness and behaviour problems. Both studies provide some indication of the kind of work-load which characterises work in a pediatric hospital setting, though the specific problems referred may be a function of the expertise of individual psychologists, rather than a reflection of the frequency of different types of problems. Thus, the fact that one hospital based psychological service receives a number of referrals for children with chronic disease needing help to overcome needle phobia may reflect the fact that an individual has developed some expertise in that area. In another setting rather more referrals may involve preparing children for radiotherapy or dealing with eating problems.

Implications for practice

Children with chronic disease

Perhaps more than anything else this review highlights the extent to which we have relied on parents' reports about their child's reactions to chronic disease, rather than involve children themselves. Although some children will undoubtedly find it difficult to talk about their experiences (and their feelings should always be considered first), it is easy to underestimate children's abilities in this respect. In addition, we shy away from situations which may be difficult for us, as interviewers, to handle. Where children have been involved more directly in work, they show considerable insight and powers of perception. Their insight, especially in terms of inferring the seriousness of disease in the absence of specific information, and keeping this information to themselves rather than worry others, has been well documented (Binger *et al.* 1969). Much of our information is based on isolated clinical cases, rather than systematic collection of data. There is some assumption that children who have chronic disease, or survive cancer, consider themselves 'special' or destined for great things. Others do not always feel so grateful.

'I lost five years of my life through that treatment' (18-year-old survivor of leukemia).

It is not surprising that this boy feels resentful about still having to come back to the clinic, and reminded that he is lucky and should feel grateful. Yet by talking only to his parents, one would get the impression that the whole family felt very positively about the way in which treatment worked. Children do not necessarily share their parents' perspective, and we need to be more aware of this. Whatever the child's physical status, parents may be grateful that the child is alive. Children may be less sure about the value of 'just being alive' when they perceive themselves to be restricted from what they would like to do and from what others can so easily do.

Talking to children also gives some insight into their experiences with growing up with a chronic disease. While parents (and medical staff) may be content to assess success in terms of academic achievement, children have other criteria. Social relationships within the school are important. Although teachers have some control over relationships in the classroom, there is little they can do in the playground, in the canteen, or on journeys to and from school. It is in these situations that children can be cruel and unfeeling. What can be more unfeeling than the boys in a school playground who called after a girl who had undergone major surgery to correct cancer in the leg;

'If you run any faster your leg will drop off...'

Healthy children

This example highlights the fact that healthy children need some education about how to respond to others, especially those with visible malformations. While some children find it helpful to discuss their condition in front of the class, others lack the ability or confidence to act in this way. Interventions which encourage healthy children to empathise with the sick child have been associated with some success (Benner & Marlow 1991; Treiber, Schramm & Mabe 1986).

Pediatricians are generally very good at understanding that chronic disease in a child affects the whole family and every individual member. What is less generally acknowledged is that the impact of the disease goes even beyond the immediate family. Few people are very sensitive as to how they interact with chronically sick or dying children. Mothers often complain that friends and neighbours discuss the child's health in the child's presence, but pretending they are not there, or deaf. The situation heightens many emotions, including relief that we are not ourselves having to deal with the disease in our own families, and fear about the consequences. As soon as the immediate crisis is over, however, children are expected to pick up their lives as if nothing has happened, and in doing so they come into contact with individuals who understand little of their situation. Teachers and other children in the school are those with whom the child is forced into most contact. Both groups have a crucial role to play in helping the child adjust to the situation and get the best out of life outside the family circle. Lack of information and fear mean that less is often achieved than should be. More routine education of the public generally should become an integral part of the psychologist's role.

Siblings

Healthy siblings remain a neglected group. The question of how to deal with healthy siblings is far from easy. Some parents feel strongly that the disease should make as little impact on the lives of their other children as possible.

'When Jo was diagnosed, we decided to keep Tom's life as normal as possible. My wife went to the hospital with Jo; I stayed home with Tom. We carried on as best we could. Each morning we would get up as we always had done and I would go to work and Tom to school. He had a big exam. coming up and we felt we owed it to him, not to spoil his chances. Now that Jo is dead, we're really glad that we did it that way. There was nothing he could have done, and now he has his life before him. There would be no point compromising his whole future.'

Others make the same decision but come to regret it.

'I left Sukey with my mother while I spent all my time in hospital with Jane. Sukey used to come and see us sometimes and she seemed happy enough, and I used to ring every night. She seemed alright when we first got home too. It was 18 months later when the trouble really started. She got very clingy, and hates me to go anywhere. She's always talking about Jane's illness; she's a real hypochondriac, always got a pain somewhere. I really regret that I left her, in retrospect, it was the worse thing I ever did.'

Decisions about how far to involve healthy siblings are often only judged with hindsight. Where siblings adjust well and show few subsequent behavioural or emotional problems, parents feel justified about their decisions. Where problems occur, parents tend to doubt their original decisions about involving the child. In reality, we do not know if the sibling's initial involvement is significant for later adjustment. In

both cases above, it is not known if the sibling involved would acknowledge the importance of these early experiences in shaping their current
behaviour. What is clear is that the issue becomes important to parents;
subsequent adjustment of healthy siblings is often attributed to the
success or otherwise of the arrangements initially made for them.

Other parents certainly make very different decisions, involving the
healthy child as far as possible. This can mean taking the child from
school in order to live with the rest of the family near the hospital where
the child is being treated. The long term impact on these siblings, in
terms of lack of academic achievement and compromised prospects, is
considerable.

Sibling relationships in all families are complex, and it is too easy for
siblings to feel resentment towards each other. Many siblings feel helped
by occasional visits to the hospital, and the opportunity to see exactly
what happens there. Others report some benefits from meeting other
siblings, and being able to discuss with them their feelings about the
changes in family relationships (Kinrade 1985).

Parents

It is not always clear how research data should best be used. For
example, having a child with chronic disease is definitely a strain on any
relationship, and can sometimes contribute to unease and ultimately
divorce. To what extent is this information useful to parents of newly
diagnosed children? Some staff clearly feel it would be useful to be
informed and therefore prepared; others prefer to limit information to
that which can definitely be expected. Yet it is a common mistake to
attribute all a family's problems to the disease in one child. Medical staff
are well aware of the potential strain that can result from looking after
a child with chronic disease, but they are rarely aware of other problems
a family may face. This can mean that they place too much emphasis on
the consequences of the disease, forgetting that difficulties with other
family members or at work can be equally important.

It is not just in the context of emotional relationships that such
dilemmas arise. Many children who are prescribed specific drugs are
known to experience side-effects in terms of mood shifts and tantrums.
Yet it is often felt wise not to inform parents who might then be highly
tuned to expect these side effects and therefore identify them anyway.
Parents who are not informed, but whose child develops such side
effects can feel very angry and cheated by medical staff, and perceive
them to be dishonest. Staff, however, justify withholding the information on the grounds that there is no point in causing anxiety unnecessarily. Decisions need to be made about when and under what
circumstances results of research need to be made available to parents.

Perhaps the answer to the question of what circumstances has to do with the kind of help which is available. Information about the possibility of behavioural side-effects associated with drugs is only really useful if accompanied by information about when the effects are most likely to be experienced and how they can be dealt with. Perhaps administering the drugs just before the child goes to bed can be strategic. If this is not possible, how can parents be advised to deal with the tantrums, both so as to help the child and to minimise the impact on the rest of the family? The extent to which parents can be helped by the opportunity to talk to other parents in the same situation cannot be overlooked. Groups specifically for this purpose are potentially useful, but may not be available at the most appropriate times. Groups of parents who have already been through similar circumstances but who are prepared to act as 24 hour counselling services to others, have a role to play.

Epilogue

There can be no disputing the improvements that have taken place in the care of sick children generally and those with chronic disease more specifically over the last few decades. Pediatric wards are more pleasant and colourful places to be. There are activities for children to do, and friends and family can visit with few restrictions. Enormous strides have been made in caring for children with previously fatal and degenerative conditions.

But these changes are not without some cost. Chronic disease invariably has some implications for the child's development. There may be some physical limitation, restricting strenuous activity. There may be some academic difficulties, reflecting interruptions in schooling or side-effects of treatments. There may be some social difficulties, again reflecting interruptions in schooling or the fact that the child spends so much more time in the company of adults rather than peers. For too long, success in treatment of chronic disease has been measured in terms of survival, with little attention paid to the more social and emotional consequences. Current theorizing in psychology which stresses the resilience and coping of many families also contributes to a view that plays down the potentially disruptive and destructive nature of surviving chronic disease. Very little research has addressed the long term consequences of chronic disease. Work that does, points to residual problems for these children, including those living with relatively mild asthma, through to long term survivors of childhood cancer.

In part, these long term difficulties are a product of society's intolerance and lack of provision of appropriate resources. The fragmentation of medical, social and educational services limits the efficacy of care provided, and confuses families. Integration of services is necessary along with changes in the threshold for referrals. There needs to be a shift from referrals during crisis, to a service organised more around the idea of prevention. Communities rarely offer any back-up services outside the hospital setting to give children the opportunities to make up for lost social and educational time while they were ill. Provision of appropriate services in the community needs to be seen as an integral part of the care of the child. However much medicine may advance to a point at which children survive serious and life-threatening conditions, it will be to no avail unless educational and psychological services make corresponding progress.

References

Abidin, R. (1990) Introduction to the special issue: The stresses of parenting. *Journal of Clinical Child Psychology, 19,* 298– 301.

Abidin, R.R. (1983) *Parenting Stress Index (PSI) – Manual.* Charlottesville, V.A.

Abidin, R.R. and Burke, W.T. (1978) *The Development of the Parenting Stress Index.* Paper presented at the annual meeting of the American Psychological Association. Toronto.

Abroms, K.I. and Kodera, T.L. (1979) Acceptance hierarchy of handicaps: Validation of Kirk's statement, 'Special Education often begins where medicine stops'. *Journal of Learning Disabilities, 12,* 15–20.

Achenbach, T. and Edelbrock, C. (1983) *Manual for the Child Behaviour Checklist and Revised Child Behaviour Profile.* Burlington, VT: University of Burlington Press.

Achenbach, T. and Edelbrock, C. (1986) *Manual for the Teacher's Report Form and Teacher Version of the Child Behaviour Profile.* Burlington: University of Vermont.

Ack, M., Miller, I. and Weil, W.B. (1961) Intelligence of children with diabetes mellitus. *Pediatrics, 25,* 764–70.

Affleck, G., Tennen, H. and Rowe, J. (1990) Mothers, fathers, and the crisis of newborn intensive care. *Infant Mental Health Journal, 11,* 12–25.

Affleck, G., Tennen, H. and Rowe, J. (1991) *Infants in Crisis: How Parents Cope with Newborn Intensive Care and its Aftermath.* New York: Springer-Verlag.

Affleck, G., Tennen, H., Allen, D. and Gershman, K. (1986) Perceived social support and maternal adaptation during the transition from hospital to home care of high risk infants. *Infant Mental Health Journal, 7,* 6–18.

Ainsworth, M.D.S., Blehar, M.C., Waters, E. and Wall, S. (1978) *Patterns of Attachment.* Hillsdale, N.J: Erlbaum.

Allan, J.C., Townley, R. and Phelan, P.D. (1974) Family response to cystic fibrosis. *Australian Pediatric Journal, 10,* 136–146.

Allen, D.A., Affleck, G., Tennen, H., McGrade, B.J. and Ratzan, S. (1984) Concerns of children with a chronic illness: A cognitive-developmental study of juvenile diabetes. *Child: Care, Health and Development, 10,* 211–218.

Allen, D.A., Tennen, H., McGrade, B.J., Affleck, G. and Ratzan, S. (1983) Parent and child perceptions of the management of juvenile diabetes. *Journal of Pediatric Psychology, 8,* 129–141.

Allen, R., Wasserman, G.A. and Seidman, S. (1990) Children with congenital anomalies: The preschool period. *Journal of Pediatric Psychology, 15,* 327–346.

Altshuler, J.L. and Ruble, D.N. (1989) Developmental changes in children's awareness of strategies for coping with uncontrollable stress. *Child Development, 60,* 1337–1349.

Anderson, B.J. (1990) Diabetes and adaptations in family systems. In C.S. Holmes (ed.) *Neuropsychological and Behavioural Aspects of Diabetes.* New York: Springer-Verlag. pp.85–101.

Anderson, B.J., Auslander, W.F., Jung, K., Miller, J.P. and Santiago, J.V. (1990) Assessing family sharing of diabetes responsibilities. *Journal of Pediatric Psychology, 15,* 477–492.

Anderson, B.J., Miller, J.P., Auslander, W.F. and Santiago, J.V. (1981) Family characteristics of diabetic adolescents: Relationships to metabolic control. *Diabetes Care, 4,* 586–594.

Anderson, H.R., Bailey, P.A., Cooper, J.A., Palmer, J.S. and West, S. (1983) Morbidity and school absence caused by asthma and wheezing illness. *Archives of Disease in Childhood, 58,* 777–784.

Andrews, S.G. (1991) Informing schools about children's chronic illnesses: Parents' Opinions. *Pediatrics, 88,* 306–311.

Antonucci, J. (1976) Attachment: A life-span concept. *Human Development, 19,* 135–152.

Appolone-Ford, C., Gibson, P. and Driefuss, F.E. (1983) (eds.) *Pediatrics: Epileptology, Classification and Management of Seizures in the Child.* Littleton, MA: PSG Publishing.

Baker, L., Rossman, B., Sargent, J., Nogueira, J. and Stanley, C.A. (1982) Family factors predict glycosylated hemoglobin (HbA) in juvenile diabetes: A prospective study. *Diabetes, 31,* (Suppl. 2), 15a.

Band, E.B. (1990) Children's coping with diabetes: Understanding the role of cognitive development. *Journal of Pediatric Psychology, 15,* 27–41.

Band, E.B. and Weisz, J.R. (1988) How to feel better when it feels bad: Children's perspectives on coping with everyday stress. *Developmental Psychology, 24,* 247–253.

Bandura, A. (1977) *Social Learning Theory.* Englewood Cliffs, New Jersey: Prentice Hall.

Banion, J.R., Miles, M.S. and Carter, M.C. (1983) Problems of mothers in management of children with diabetes. *Diabetes Care, 6,* 548–551.

Bank, S. and Kahn, M. (1975) Sisterhood-brotherhood is powerful: Sibling sub-systems in family therapy. *Family Processes, 14,* 311–339.

Barbarin, O.A., Hughes, D. and Chesler, M.A. (1985) Stress, coping, and marital functioning among parents of children with cancer. *Journal of Marriage and the Family, 47,* 473–480.

Barrett, A.J. and Gordon-Smith, E.C. (1983) *Bone Marrow Transplantation: A Review.* Oxford: Medicine Publishing Foundation.

Baruch, G.K. and Barnett, R.C. (1986) Fathers' participation in family work and children's sex-role attitudes. *Child Development, 57,* 1210–1223.

Baumrind, D. (1978) Parental disciplinary patterns and social competence in children. *Youth and Society,* March, 237–276.

Beck, A.T. (1967) *Depression: Clinical, Experimental, and Theoretical Aspects*. New York: Harper and Row.

Bellah, R.N., Madsen, R., Sullivan, W.M., Swidler, A. and Tipton, S.M. (1985) *Habits of the Heart: Individuation and Commitment in American Life*. New York: Harper and Row.

Belsky, J. and Isabella, R. (1988) Maternal, infant and social-contextual determinants of attachment security. In J. Belsky and T. Nezworski (eds.) *Clinical Implications of Attachment*. Hillsdale, N.J.: Erlbaum (pp.41–94).

Bendell, R.D., Culbertson, J.C., Skelton, R.L. and Carter, B.D. (1986) Interrupted infantile copnea: Impact in early development. *Journal of Clinical Child Psychology, 15*, 304–310.

Benner, A.E. and Marlow, L.S. (1991) The effect of a workshop on childhood cancer on students' knowledge and desire to interact with a classmate with cancer. *Childrens' Health Care, 20*, 101–107.

Bevis, M. and Taylor, B. (1990) What do school teachers know about asthma? *Archives of Disease in Childhood, 65*, 622–625.

Bibace, R. and Walsh, M.E. (1981) Children's conceptions of illness. In R. Bibace and M.E. Walsh (eds.) *New Directions for Child Development: No. 14 Children's Conceptions of Health, Illness and Bodily Functions*. San Francisco: Jossey-Bass.

Binger, C.M., Ablin, A.R., Feuerstein, R.C., Kushner, J.H., Roger, S. and Mikkelson, C. (1969) Childhood leukemia: Emotional impact on patient and family. *New England Journal of Medicine, 280*, 414–418.

Birenbaum, L.K. (1970) Family coping with childhood cancer. *The Hospice Journal, 6*, 17–33.

Bloch, C.A., Clemmons, P.S. and Sperling, M.A. (1987) Puberty decreases insulin sensitivity. *Journal of Pediatrics, 110*, 481–487.

Bloch, J.H. (1981) The child-rearing practices report (CRPR): A set of questions for the description of parental socialization attitudes and values. Unpublished manuscript, Institute of Human Development, University of California, Berkeley.

Bloch, J.H., Block, J. and Morrison, A. (1981) Parental agreement–disagreement on child-rearing orientations and gender-related personality correlates in children. *Child Development, 52*, 965–974.

Block, J. and Block, J. (1980) The role of ego-control and ego-resiliency in the organization of behaviour. In W.A. Collins (ed.) *Minnesota Symposium on Child Psychology* (Vol. 13) (pp.39–101). Hillsdale, N.J: Erlbaum.

Bloomfield, S. and Farquhar, J.W. (1990) Is a specialist pediatric diabetic clinic better? *Archives of Disease in Childhood, 65*, 139–140.

Blount, R.L., Corbin, S.H., Sturgess, J.W., Wolfe, V.V., Prater, J.M. and James, L.D. (1989) The relationship between adult's behaviour and child coping and distress during BMA/LP procedures: A sequential analysis. *Behaviour Therapy, 20*, 585–601.

Bluebond-Langner, M. (1977) Meanings of death to children. In H. Feifel (ed.) *New Meanings of Death*. New York: McGraw-Hill (pp.46–66).

Bluebond-Langner, M., Perkel, D., Goertzel, T., Nelson, K. and McGeary, J. (1990) Children's knowledge of cancer and its treatment. Impact of an oncology camp experience. *Journal of Pediatrics, 116,* 207–213.

Bobrow, E.S., AvEuskin, T.W. and Siller, J. (1985) Mother–daughter interaction and adherence to diabetes regimens. *Diabetes Care, 8,* 145–156.

Boer, F. (1990) *Sibling Relationships in Middle Childhood.* Leiden: DSWO University of Leiden Press.

Boggs, S.R., Graham-Pole, J. and Miller, E.M. (1991) Life- threatening illness and invasive treatment: The future of life assessment and research in pediatric oncology. In J.H. Johnson and S. Bennett-Johnson (eds.) *Advances in Child Health Psychology.* Gainesville: University of Florida Press. (pp.353–361).

Bowlby, J. (1969) *Attachment and Loss* (Vol. 1) New York: Basic Books.

Boyle, I.R., de Sant' Aguese, P., Sack, S., Millican, F. and Kukczycki, L.L. (1976) Emotional adjustment of adolescents and young adults with cystic fibrosis. *Journal of Pediatrics, 88,* 318–326.

Bradbury, J.A. and Smith, C.W. (1983) An assessment of the diabetic knowledge of school teachers. *Archives of Disease in Childhood, 58,* 692–696.

Bregani, P., Della Porta, V., Carbonne, A., Ongari, B. and di Natale, B. (1979) Attitudes of juvenile diabetics and their families towards diabetic regimen. *Pediatric and Adolescent Endocrinology, 7,* 159–163.

Breslau, N. and Marshall, S. (1985) Psychiatric disorder in children with physical disabilities. *Journal of the American Academy of Child Psychiatry, 24,* 87–94.

Breslau, N., Staruch, K.S. and Mortimer, E.A. Jnr. (1982) Psychological distress in mothers of disabled children. *American Journal of Diseases of Children, 136,* 682–686.

Breslau, N., Weitzman, M. and Messenger, K. (1981) Psychologic functioning of siblings of disabled children. *Pediatrics, 67,* 344–353.

Bretherton, I. and Waters, E. (1985) Growing pains in attachment theory and research. *Monograms of the Society of Research in Child Development, 50,* (1–2, Serial No. 209).

Brewer, E.U., McPherson, M. and Masrab, P.R. (1989) Family centred, community based coordinated care for children with special health care needs. *Pediatrics, 83,* 1055–1060.

Briggs, D. (1985) The impact on a family of having a newborn baby hospitalized in a newborn intensive care unit. Unpublished doctoral disseration. Brandeis University, Waltham, M.A.

Bronfenbrenner, W. (1979) *The Ecology of Human Development.* Cambridge, MA: Harvard University Press.

Buchanan, D.C., La Barbara, C.J., Roelofs, R. and Olson, W. (1979) Reactions of families with children with Duchene muscular dystrophy. *General Hospital Psychiatry, 1,* 262–269.

Burstein, S. and Meichenbaum, D. (1979) The work of worrying in children undergoing surgery. *Journal of Abnormal Child Psychology, 7,* 121–131.

Burton, L. (1975) *The Family Life of Sick Children.* London: Routledge and Kegan Paul.

Bush, J.P., Melamed, B.G., Sheras, P.J. and Greenbaum, P.E. (1986) Mother–child patterns of coping with anticipatory medical stress. *Health Psychology, 5,* 137–157.

Bywater, E. (1981) Adolescents with cystic fibrosis: Psychosocial adjustment. *Archives of Disease in Childhood, 56,* 538–543.

Cadman, D., Boyle, M. and Offord, D.R. (1988) The Ontario Child Health Study: Social adjustment and mental health of siblings of children with chronic health problems. *Journal of Developmental and Behavioural Pediatrics, 9,* 117–121.

Cadman, D., Boyle, M., Szatmari, P., Offord, D.R. (1987) Chronic illness, disability and mental and social well-being: Findings of the Ontario Child Health Study. *Pediatrics, 79,* 805–813.

Cadman, D., Rosenbaum, P., Boyle, M. and Offord, D. (1991) Children with chronic illness: Family and parent demographic characteristics and psychosocial adjustment. *Pediatrics, 87,* 884–889.

Cain, A., Fast, I. and Erickson, M. (1964) Children's disturbed reactions to the death of a sibling. *American Journal of Orthopsychiatry, 34,* 741–752.

Cairns, N. and Lanskey, S.B. (1980) MMPI Indicators of stress and marital discord among parents of children with chronic illness. *Death Education, 4,* 29–42.

Cairns, N., Clark, G., Smith, S. and Lansky, S. (1979) Adaptation of siblings to childhood malignancy. *Journal of Pediatrics, 95,* 484–487.

Cappelli, M., MacDonald, N.E. and McGrath, P.J. (1989) Assessment of readiness to transfer to adult care for adolescents with cystic fibrosis. *Children's Health Care, 1989, 18,* 218–224.

Cappelli, M., McGrath, P.J., MacDonald, N.E., Katsamis, J. and Lascellas, M. (1989) Parental care and overprotection of children with cystic fibrosis. *British Journal of Medical Psychology, 62,* 281–289.

Carpenter, P.J. and Sahler, O.J.Z. (1991) Sibling perception and adaptation to childhood cancer: Conceptual and methodological considerations. In J.H. Johnson and S.B. Johnson (eds.) *Advances in Child Health Psychology.* Gainesville: University of Florida Press.

Carr, J., Pearson, A. and Halliwell, H. (1983) The effect of disability on family life. *Zeitschrift fur kinderchirurgie, 38,* Supp. II, 103–106.

Carr-Gregg, M. and White, L. (1987) Siblings of paediatric cancer patients: A population at risk. *Medical and Paediatric Oncology, 15,* 62–68.

Carr-Gregg, M., White, L., O'Gorman-Hughes, D.W. and Vowells, M. (1985) Psychological functioning in pediatric cancer patients. (Meeting Abstract) *Medical Pediatric Oncology, 3,* 143.

Carroll, G., Massarelli, E., Opzcomer, A., Pekeles, G., Pedneault, M., Frappier, J. and Onetto, N. (1983) Adolescents with chronic disease: Are they receiving comprehensive health care? *Journal of Adolescent Health Care, 4,* 261–265.

Carver, C.S., Scheier, M.F. and Weintraub, J.K. (1989) Assessing coping strategies: A theoretically based approach. *Journal of Personality and Social Psychology, 56,* 267–283.

Cerreto, M.C. (1986) Developmental issues in chronic illness: Implications and applications. *Topics in Early Childhood Special Education, 5,* 23–35.

Cerreto, M.C. and Travis, L.B. (1984) Implications of psychological and family factors in the treatment of diabetes. *Pediatric Clinics of North America, 31,* 689–690.

Challen, A.H., Davies, A.S., Williams, R.J.W., Haslum, M.N. and Baum, J.D. (1988) Measuring psychological adaptation to diabetes in adolescence. *Diabetic Medicine, 5,* 739–746.

Chaney, J.M. and Peterson, L. (1989) Family variables and disease management in juvenile rheumatoid arthritis. *Journal of Pediatric Psychology, 14,* 389–403.

Charlop, M.H., Parrish, J.M., Fenton, L.R. and Cataldo, M.F. (1987) Evaluation of hospital-based outpatient pediatric psychology services. *Journal of Pediatric Psychology, 12,* 485–503.

Charlton, A., Larcombe, I.J., Meller, S.T., Morris Jones, P.H., Mott, M.G., Pottan, M.W., Tranmer, M.D. and Walker, J.J.P. (1991) Absence from school related to cancer and other chronic conditions. *Archives of Disease in Childhood, 66,* 1217–1222.

Chesler, M.A., Paris, J. and Barbarin, O.A. (1986) 'Telling' the child with cancer: Parental choices to share information with ill children. *Journal of Pediatric Psychology, 11,* 497–516.

Christiaanse, M.E., Lavigne, J.V. and Lerner, C.V. (1989) Psychological aspects of compliance in children and adolescents with asthma. *Developmental and Behavioural Pediatrics, 10,* 75–80.

Circerrelli, V.G. (1982) Sibling influence throughout the life-span. In M. Lamb, and B. Sutton-Smith (eds.) *Sibling Relationships. Their Nature and Significance Across the Life-Span.* Hillsdale, N.J.: Erlbaum.

Claflin, C.J. and Barbarin, O.A. (1991) Does 'telling' less protect more? Relationships among age, information disclosure, and what children with cancer see and feel. *Journal of Pediatric Psychology, 16,* 169–192.

Cleveland, D. and Miller, N. (1977) Attitudes and life commitment of older siblings of mentally retarded adults: An exploratory study. *Mental Retardation, 3,* 38–41.

Close, H., Davies, A.G., Price, D.A. and Goodyer, I.M. (1986) Emotional difficulties in diabetes mellitus. *Archives of Disease in Childhood, 61,* 337–340.

Cluss, and Epstein, (1985) Effect of compliance for chronic asthmatic children. *Journal of Consulting and Clinical Psychology, 52,* 909–910.

Coddington, R. (1972) The significance of life-events as etiological factors in the disease of children: I and II. *Psychosomatic Research, 16,* 205–215.

Cohen, S., Friedrich, W.N., Copeland, D.R. and Pendergrass, T.W. (1989) Instruments to measure parent–child communication regarding pediatric cancer. *Children's Health Care, 18,* 142–145.

Cohen, S. and Parmelee, A. (1983) Prediction of five-year Stamford Binet scores in preterm infants. *Child Development, 54,* 1242–1253.

Collier, B.N. and Etzwiler, D. D. (1971) Comparative study of diabetes knowledge among juvenile diabetes and their parents. *Diabetes, 20,* 51–57.

Compas, B.E. (1987) Coping with stress during childhood and adolescence. *Psychological Bulletin, 101,* 393–403.

Compas, B.E., Malcarne, V.L. and Fondacaro, K.M. (1988) Coping with stressful events in older children and young adolescents. *Journal of Consulting and Clinical Psychology, 56,* 405–411.

Compas, B.E., Worsham, N.L. and Ey, S. (1992) Conceptual and developmental issues in children's coping with stress. In A.M., La Greca, L.J. Siegel, J.L. Wallander and C.E. Walker (eds.) *Stress and Coping in Child Health.* New York: The Guilford Press. (pp.7–24).

Cook, J. (1984) Influence of gender on the problems of parents of fatally ill children. *Journal of Psychosocial Oncology, 2,* 71–91.

Cousens, P., Waters, B., Said, J. and Stevens, M. (1988) Cognitive effects of cranial irradiation in leukemia: A survey and meta-analysis. *Journal of Child Psychology and Psychiatry, 29,* 839–852.

Cowen, L., Corey, M., Keenan, N., Simmons, R., Arndt, E. and Levison, H. (1985) Family adaptation and psychosocial adjustment to cystic fibrosis in the preschool child. *Social Science and Medicine, 20,* 553–560.

Cowen, L., Corey, M., Simmons, R., Keenan, N., Robertson, J. and Levison, H. (1984) Growing older with cystic fibrosis: Psychologic adjustment of patients over 16 years old. *Psychosomatic Medicine, 46,* 363–376.

Cox, M.J., Owen, M.T., Henderson, V.K., and Margand, N.A. (1992) Prediction of infant–father and infant–mother attachment. *Developmental Psychology, 28,* 474–483.

Coyne, J.C., Wortman, C.B. and Lehman, D.R. (1988) The other side of support: Emotional overinvolvement and miscarried helping. In B.H. Gottlieb (ed.) *Marshaling Social Support: Formats, Processes and Effects.* Newbury Park, CA: Sage, (pp.305–330).

Craft, M. (1985) Responses in siblings of hospitalized children (Doctoral dissertation, University of Iowa).

Craft, M.J. and Craft, J.L. (1989) Perceived changes in siblings of hospitilized children: A comparison of sibling and parent reports. *Children's Health Care, 18,* 42–48.

Crain, A., Sussman, M. and Weill, W. Jr. (1966) Effects of a diabetic child on marital integration and related measures of family functioning. *Journal of Health and Human Behaviour, 7,* 122–127.

Crider, C. (1981) Children's concepts of the body interior. In R. Bibace and M. Walsh (eds.) *Children's Conceptions of Health, illness and Bodily Functions.* San Francisco: Jossey-Bass.

Crocker, A. (1981) The involvement of siblings of children with handicaps. In A. Milunsky (ed.) *Coping with Crisis and Handicap.* New York: Plenum.

Cull, A. (1991) Staff support in medical oncology: A problem-solving approach. *Psychology and Health, 5,* 129–136.

Cummings, S.T. (1976) The impact of the child's deficiency on the father: A study of fathers of mentally retarded and chronically ill children. *American Journal of Orthopsychiatry, 46,* 246–255.

Cummings, S.T., Bayley, H.C. and Rie, H.E. (1966) Effects of the child's deficiency on the mother: A study of mothers of mentally retarded, chronically ill, and neurotic children. *American Journal of Orthopsychiatry, 36,* 595–608.

Cunningham, C. Betsa, N. and Gross, S. (1985) Sibling groups: Interaction with siblings of oncology patients. *American Journal of Pediatric Hematology and Oncology, 3,* 135–139.

Curry, S.L. and Russ, S.W. (1985) Identifying coping strategies in children. *Journal of Clinical Child Psychology, 14,* 61–69.

Daniels, D., Dunn, J., Furstenberg, F. and Plomin, R. (1985) Environmental differences within the family and adjustment differences within pairs of adolescent siblings. *Child Development, 56,* 764–774.

Daniels, D., Miller, J.J., Billings, A.H. and Moos, R.H. (1986) Psychosocial functioning of siblings of children with rheumatic disease. *Journal of Pediatrics, 109,* 379–383.

Darke, P. and Goldberg, S. Hello-goodbye: A method for assessing father–infant interaction. (unpublished manuscript)

Davies, W.H., Noll, R.B., Stefano, L., Bukowski, W.M. and Kulkarni, R. (1991) Differences in the child-rearing practices of parents of children with cancer and controls: The perpectives of parents and professionals. *Journal of Pediatric Psychology, 16,* 295–306.

Davis, P.B. and May, J.E. (1991) Involving fathers in early intervention and family support programs: Issues and strategies. *Childrens' Health Care, 20,* 87–92.

Deasey-Spinetta, P. Spinetta, J.J. and Oxman, J.B. (1988) The relationship between learning deficits and social adaptation in children with leukemia. *Journal of Psychosocial Oncology, 6,* 109–121.

Deasy-Spinetta, P. and Spinetta, J.J. (1980) The child with cancer in school: Teacher's appraisal. *American Journal of Pediatric Hematology and Oncology, 2,* 89–94.

DeMaso, D.R., Campis, L.K., Wypij, D., Bertram, S., Lipshitz, M. and Freed, M. (1991) The impact of maternal perceptions and medical severity on the adjustment of children with congenital heart disease. *Journal of Pediatric Psychology, 16,* 137–150.

Denning, R., Gluckson, M.M. and Mohr, I. (1976) Psychological and social aspects of cystic fibrosis. In J.A. Mangos and R.C. Talamo (eds.) *Cystic Fibrosis – Projections into the Future.* New York: Stratton International Medical Book Corporation.

Dikmen, S., Mathews, C.G. and Harley, J.P. (1975) The effect of early vs. late onset of major motor epilepsy upon cognitive intellectual performance. *Epilepsia, 16,* 73–81.

Dishion, T. (1986) *Peer Rejection.* Seminar to Oregon Learning Centre.

DiVitto, B. and Goldberg, S. (1979) The effects of newborn medical status on early parent-infant interaction. In T. Field, A. Sostek and S. Goldberg (eds.) *Infants Born at Risk.* New York: Spectrum (pp.311–332).

Dolgin, M.J. and Katz, E.R. (1988) Conditioned aversions in pediatric cancer patients receiving chemotherapy. *Journal of Developmental and Behavioural Pediatrics, 9,* 82–85.

Dolgin, M.J., Phipps, S., Harow, E. and Zeltzer, L.K. (1990) Parental management of fear in chronically ill and healthy children. *Journal of Pediatric Psychology, 15,* 733–744.

Donnelly, J.E., Donnelly, W.J. and Thong, Y.H. (1987) Parental perceptions and attitudes toward asthma and its treatment: a controlled study. *Social Science and Medicine, 24,* 431–437.

Doyle, B.J. and Ware, J.E. (1977) Physician conduct and other factors that affect consumer satisfaction with medical care. *Journal of Medical Education, 52,* 793–801.

Doyle, J.A. (1983) *The Male Experience.* Dubuque, Iowa: Wm. C. Brown Co. Publishers.

Drash, A.L. (1979) The child with diabetes. In B. Hamburg, L. Lipsett, G. Inoff and A. Drash (eds.) *Behavioural and Psychosocial Issues in Diabetes* U.S. Department of Health and Human Service: NIH Publication No. 80–1993 (pp.33–42).

Drotar, D. (1978) Psychological research in pediatric settings: Lessons from the field. *Journal of Pediatric Psychology, 19,* 63–79.

Drotar, D. and Crawford, P. (1985) Psychological adaptation of siblings of chronically ill children: Research and practice implications. *Developmental and Behavioural Pediatrics, 6,* 355–362.

Drotar, D., Baskieweicz, A., Irvin, N., Kennell, J. and Klaus, M. (1975) The adaptation of parents to the birth of an infant with a congenital malformation: A hypothetical model. *Pediatrics, 6,* 710–717.

Drotar, D., Crawford, P. and Bush, M. (1984) The family context of childhood chronic illness: Implications for psychosocial intervention. In M.G. Eisenberg, L.C. Sutkin and M.A. Jansen (eds.) *Chronic Illness and Disability Throughout the Life-span: Effects on Self and Family.* New York: Springer (pp.103–129).

Dunbar, H.F. (1954) *Emotions and Bodily Changes.* New York: Columbia University Press.

Dunn, J. (1987) Introduction. In F.F. Schachter and R.K. Stone (eds.) Practical concerns about siblings: Bridging the research-practice gap. *Journal of Children in Contemporary Society, 19,* 1–11.

Dunn, J. (1988) Sibling influences on childhood development. *Journal of Child Psychology and Psychiatry, 29,* 119–128.

Dunn, J. and McGuire, S. (1992) Sibling and peer relationships in childhood. *Journal of Child Psychology and Psychiatry, 33,* 67–106.

Dunn, J. and Munn, P. (1986) Siblings and the development of prosocial behaviour. *International Journal of Behavioural Development, 9,* 265–284.

Dunn-Geier, J., McGrath, P., Rourke, B.P., Latter, J. and D'Astons, J. (1986) Adolescent chronic pain: The ability to cope. *Pain, 26,* 23–32.

Easterbrooks, A. and Emde, R. (1988) Marital and parent–child relationships: The role of affect in the family system. In R. Hinde and J. Stevenson-Hinde (eds.)

Relationships Within Families: Mutual Influences (pp.104–141). Oxford: Oxford University Press.

Easterbrooks, M.A. and Goldberg, W. (1984) Effects of early maternal employment on toddlers, mothers and fathers. *Developmental Psychology, 25,* 774–783.

Eccles, J.S. and Midgley, C. (1989) Stage 1 environment fit: Developmentally appropriate classrooms for early adolescents. In R. Ames and C. Ames (eds.) *Research on Motivation in Education* (Vol. 3 pp.130–181). San Diego, California: Academic Press.

Editorial (1972) Age limits of pediatrics. *Pediatrics, 49,* 463.

Egeland, B. and Sroufe, L.A. (1981) Developmental sequelae of maltreatment in infancy. In R. Rizley and D. Cicchetti (eds.) *Developmental Perspectives in Child and Treatment.* San Francisco: Jossey-Bass (pp.77–92).

Eiser, C. (1980) How leukemia affects a child's schooling. *British Journal of Social and Clinical Psychology, 19,* 365–368.

Eiser, C. (1985) *The Psychology of Childhood Illness.* New York: Springer-Verlag.

Eiser, C. (1989) Children's understanding of illness: A critique of the 'stage' approach. *Psychology and Health, 3,* 93–101.

Eiser, C. (1990) Psychological effects of chronic disease. *Journal of Child Psychology and Psychiatry, 31,* 85–98.

Eiser, C. (1991) Cognitive deficits in children treated for leukemia. *Archives of Disease in Childhood, 66,* 164–168.

Eiser, C. and Havermans, T. (1992) Mothers' and fathers' coping with chronic childhood disease. *Psychology and Health, 7,* 249–257.

Eiser, C. and Lansdown, R. (1977) A retrospective study of intellectual development in children treated for acute lymphoblastic leukemia. *Archives of Disease in Childhood, 52,* 525–529.

Eiser, C. and Patterson, D. (1983) Slugs and snails and puppy-dog tails: Children's ideas about the insides of their bodies. *Child: Care, Health and Development, 9,* 233–240.

Eiser, C. and Town, C. (1987) Teachers' concerns about chronically sick children. Implications for pediatricians. *Developmental Medicine and Child Neurology, 29,* 56–63.

Eiser, C., Eiser, J.R., Town, C. and Tripp, J. (1991a) Discipline strategies and parental perceptions of pre-school children with asthma. *British Journal of Medical Psychology, 64,* 45–53.

Eiser, C., Eiser, J.R., Town, C. and Tripp, J. (1991b) Severity of asthma and parental discipline practices. *Patient Education and Counselling, 17,* 227–233.

Eiser, C., Flynn, M., Green, E., Havermans, T., Kirby, R., Sandeman, D. and Tooke, J.E. (1992) Coming of age with diabetes: Patients' view of a clinic for under-25 year olds. *Diabetic Medicine, 10,* 285–289.

Eiser, C., Havermans, T. and Casas, R. (1993) Healthy children's understanding of their blood: Implications for explaining leukemia to children. *British Journal of Educational Psychology, 63,* 528–537.

Eiser, C., Havermans, T. and Eiser, J.R. (1995) Parents attributions about childhood cancer: Implications for relationships with medical staff. *Child Care, Health and Development, 21,* 31–42.

Eiser, C., Havermans, T., Pancer, M. and Eiser, J.R. (1992) Adjustment to chronic disease in relation to age and gender: Mothers' and fathers' reports of their children's behaviour. *Journal of Pediatric Psychology*, 17, 261–276.

Eiser, C., Patterson, D. and Town, R. (1985) Knowledge of diabetes and implications for self-care. *Diabetic Medicine*, 2, 288–291.

Eiser, J.R., Morgan, M., Gammage, P., Brooks, N. and Kirby, R. (1991) Adolescent health behaviour and similarity-attraction: Friends share smoking habits (really), but much else besides. *British Journal of Social Psychology*, 30, 339–348.

Elkind, D. (1967) Egocentrism in adolescence. *Child Development*, 38, 1025–1034.

Elkins, P.D. and Roberts, M.C. (1983) Psychosocial preparation for pediatric hospitalization. *Clinical Psychology Review*, 3, 275–295.

Ellsworth, R.B. (1979) *CAAP Scale: The Measurement of Child and Adolescent Adjustment*. Roanoke, VA: Institute for Program Evaluation.

Erikson, E.H. (1959) Identity and the life-cycle. *Psychological Issues*, 1, 18–164.

Erikson, E.H. (1964) *Childhood and Society*. New York: Norton.

Escalona, S. (1953) Emotional development in the first year of life. In M.J. Senn (ed.) *Problems of Infancy and Childhood*. New York: Foundation Press.

Faust, J. and Melamed, B.G. (1984) Influence of arousal, previous experience, and age on surgery preparation of same day of surgery and in-hospital pediatric patients. *Journal of Consulting and Clinical Psychology*, 52, 359–365.

Faust, J., Olson, R. and Rodriguez, H. (1991) Same day surgery preparation: Reduction of pediatric patient arousal and distress through participant modeling. *Journal of Consulting and Clinical Psychology*, 59, 475–478.

Feeman, D.J. and Hagen, J.W. (1990) Effect of childhood chronic illness on families. *Social Work in Health Care*, 14, 37–53.

Fehrenbach, A.M.B. and Peterson, L. (1989) Parental problem-solving skills, stress, and dietary compliance in phenylketonuria. *Journal of Consulting and Clinical Psychology*, 57, 237–241.

Feldman, F.C. (1980) *Work and Cancer Health Histories: Work Expectations and Experiences of Youth with Cancer Histories (Ages 13–23)*. Oakland, California: America Cancer Society.

Feldman, S.S. and Quatman, T. (1988) Factors influencing age expectations for adolescent autonomy. *Journal of Early Adolescence*, 8, 325–343.

Ferguson, B.F. (1979) Preparing young children for hospitalization: A comparison of two methods. *Pediatrics*, 65, 656–664.

Ferrari, M. (1984) Chronic illness: Psychosocial effects on siblings – 1. Chronically ill boys. *Journal of Child Psychology and Psychiatry*, 25, 459–476.

Ferrari, M. (1987) The diabetic child and well sibling: Risks to the well child's self-concept. *Children's Health Care*, 15, 141–147.

Field, T. (1977) Effects of early separation, interactive deficits, and experimental manipulation mother-infant interaction. *Child Development*, 48, 763–771.

Field, T., Sostek, A., Goldberg, S. and Schuman, H. (1979) (eds.) *Infants Born at Risk: Behaviour and Development*. New York: Medical and Scientific Books.

Fincham, F. (1985) Attributions in close relationships. In J.H. Harvey and G. Weary (eds.) *Attribution: Basic Issues and Applications*. New York: Academic Press (pp.203–234).

Fischer-Fay, A., Goldberg, S., Simmons, R. and Levison, H. (1988) Chronic illness and infant–mother attachment: Cystic fibrosis. *Journal of Developmental and Behavioural Pediatrics, 9*, 266–270.

Fitzpatrick, M.A. (1984) A typological approach to marital interaction: Recent theory and research. In L. Berkowitz (ed.) *Advances in Experimental Social Psychology*, Vol. 18. Orlando, Florida: Academic Press (pp.1–47).

Fitzpatrick, M.A. (1990) Models of marital interaction. In H. Giles and W.P. Robinson (eds.) *Handbook of Language and Social Psychology*. Chichester, UK: Wiley. (pp.433–450).

Fobair, P., Hoppe, R.T., Bloom, J., Cox, R., Varghese, A. and Spiegel, D. (1986) Psychosocial problems among survivors of Hodgkin's disease. *Journal of Clinical Oncology, 4*, 805–814.

Fowler, M.G., Johnson, M.P. and Atkinson, S.S. (1985) School achievement and absence in children with chronic health conditions. *Journal of Pediatrics, 106*, 683–687.

Freeston, B. (1971) An enquiry into the effect of a spina bifida child upon the family. *Developmental Medicine and Child Neurology, 13*, 456–461.

Friedman, I.M. and Litt, N.F. (1986) Promoting adolescents' compliance with therapeutic regimen. *Pediatric Clinics of North America, 33*, 955–973.

Friedrich, W.N. (1979) Predictors of coping behaviour of mothers of handicapped children. *Journal of Consulting and Clinical Psychology, 47*, 1140–1141.

Gardner, G.G., August, C.S. and Githens, J. (1977) Psychological issues in bone-marrow transplantation. *Pediatrics, 60*, 625–631.

Garmezy, N., Masten, A.S. and Tellegen, A. (1984) The study of stress and competence in children: A building block for developmental psychopathology. *Child Development, 55*, 97–111.

Gath, A. (1974) Sibling reactions to mental handicap: A comparison of the brothers and sisters of mongol children. *Journal of Child Psychology and Psychiatry, 15*, 187–198.

Gayton, W.F., Friedman, S.B., Tavormina, J.F. and Tucker, F. (1977) Children with cystic fibrosis. I. Psychological test findings of patients, siblings and parents. *Pediatrics, 59*, 888–894.

Gellman, R. and Baillargeon, R. (1983) Review of some Piagetian concepts. In J.H. Flavell and E.M. Markman (eds.) *Handbook of Child Psychology, Vol. 111, Cognitive Development*. New York: Wiley.

Gil, K., Williams, D., Thompson, R. and Kinney, T. (1992) Sick cell disease in children and adolescents: The relation of child and parent pain coping strategies to adjustment. *Journal of Pediatric Psychology, 16*, 643–664.

Gillon, J.E. (1972) Family stresses when a child has congenital heart disease. *Maternal–Child Nursing Journal, 1*, 265–272.

Glasgow, R.E., McCaul, K.D. and Schafer, L.C. (1987) Self-care behaviours and glycemia control in type 1 diabetes. *Journal of Chronic Disease, 40*, 399–417.

Gogan, J.C., O'Malley, T.E. and Foster, D.J. (1977) Treating the pediatric cancer patient: A review. *Journal of Pediatric Psychology, 2,* 42–48.

Goldberg, S. (1978) Premature birth: Consequences for the parent- infant relationship. *American Scientist, 67,* 214–220.

Goldberg, S. (1982) Some biological aspects of early parent–infant interaction. In S.G. Moore and C.G. Cooper (eds.) *The Young Child: Reviews of Research.* Washington, D.C.: National Association for the Education of Young Children.

Goldberg, S. (1988) Risk factors in infant–mother attachment. *Canadian Journal of Psychology, 42,* 173–188.

Goldberg, S. and DiVitto, B. (1983) *Born Too Soon: Preterm Birth and Early Development.* San Fancisco, CA: W.H. Freeman.

Goldberg, S., Morris, P., Simmons, R.J., Fowler, R.S. and Levison, H. (1990) Chronic illness in infancy and parenting stress: A comparison of three disease groups. *Journal of Pediatric Psychology, 15,* 347–358.

Goldberg, S., Perrotta, M., Minde, K. and Corter, C. (1986) Maternal behaviour and attachment in low birth weight twins and singletons. *Child Development, 57,* 34–46.

Goldberg, S., Simmons, R.J., Newman, J., Campbell, K. and Fowler, R.S. (1991) Congenital heart disease, parental stress, and infant-mother relationships. *Journal of Pediatrics, 119,* 661–666.

Goldberg, S., Washington, J., Morris, P., Fischer-Fay, A. and Simmons, R.J. (1990) Early diagnosed chronic illness and mother–child relationships in the first two years. *Canadian Journal of Psychiatry, 35,* 726–733.

Gonder-Frederick, L., Clarke, W.L., and Snyder, A. (1987) Ability to perceive hypo- and hyper-glycemia by IDDM children and their parents. *Diabetes, 36,* 108A (Abstract 429).

Gonzales, J.C., Routh, D.K., Saab, P.G., Armstrong, F.D., Shifman, L., Guerra, E. and Fawcett, N. (1989) Effects of parent presence on children's reactions to injections: behavioural, physiological and subjective aspects. *Journal of Pediatric Psychology, 14,* 449–462.

Goodnow, J.J. (1988) Parents' ideas, actions, and feelings: Models and methods from developmental and social psychology. *Child Development, 59,* 296–320.

Gordon-Walker, J. and Manion, I. (1991) Marital interactions and family coping in pediatric chronic illness: Assessment of needs. Paper presented at the Third Florida Conference on Child Health Psychology, Gainesville, Florida.

Gortmaker, S.L. (1985) Demography of chronic childhood diseases. In N. Hobbs and J.M. Perrin (eds.) *Issues in the Care of Children with Chronic Illness.* San Francisco: Jossey-Bass.

Gortmaker, S.L., Walker, D.K., Weitzman, H. and Sobol, A.M. (1990) Chronic conditions, socioeconomic risks, and behavioural problems in children and adolescents. *Pediatrics, 85,* 267–276.

Goslin, E.R. (1978) Hospitilization as a life-crisis for the preschool child: A critical review. *Journal of Community Health, 23,* 321–346.

Green, D.M., Zevon, M.A. and Hall, B. (1991) Achievement of life goals by adult survivors of modern treatment for childhood cancer. *Cancer, 67,* 206–213.

Greenberger, E. and Goldberg, U.A. (1989) Work, parenting and the socialization of children. *Developmental Psychology, 25,* 22–35.

Greene, P. (1975) The child with leukemia in the classroom. *American Journal of Nursing, 75,* 86–87.

Grey, M.J., Genel, M. and Tamborlane, W.V. (1980) Psychological adjustment in latency-aged diabetics: Determinants and relationship to control. *Pediatrics, 65,* 69–73.

Gross, A.M., Stern, R.M., Levin, R.B., Dale, J. and Wojnilower, D.A. (1983) The effect of mother–child separation on the behaviour of children experiencing a diagnostic medical procedure. *Journal of Consulting and Clinical Psychology, 51,* 783–785.

Grossman, F.K. (1972) *Mothers and Sisters of Retarded Children: An Exploratory Story.* Syrccuse: Syrccuse University Press.

Grossman, H.Y., Brink, S. and Hauser, S.T. (1987) Self-efficacy in adolescent girls and boys with insulin-dependent diabetes mellitus. *Diabetes Care, 10,* 324–327.

Gudersmith, S. (1975) Mothers' reports of early experiences of infants with congenital heart disease. *Maternal-Child Nursing Journal, 4,* 155–164.

Hagen, J.W., Anderson, B.J., and Barclay, C.R. (1986) Issues in research on the young chronically ill child. *Topics in Early Childhood Special Education, 5,* 49–57.

Hagen, J.W., Barclay, C.R., Anderson, B.J., Feeman, D.J., Segal, S.S., Bacon, G. and Goldstein, G.W. (1990) Intellective functioning and strategy use in children with insulin dependent diabetes mellitus. *Child Development, 61,* 1714–1727.

Haggerty, R.J. (1988) Behavioural Pediatrics: A time for research. *Pediatrics, 81,* 179–185.

Hall, G.S. (1904) *Adolescence: In Psychology and its Relations to Physiology, Anthropology, Sociology, Sex, Crime, Religion and Education.* New York: Appleton.

Hamlett, K.W., Pellegrini, D.S. and Katz, K.S. (1992) Childhood chronic illness as a family stressor. *Journal of Pediatric Psychology, 17,* 33–47.

Hanson, C.L., Henggeler, S.W. and Burghen, G.A. (1987) Model of associations between psychological variables and health- outcome measures of adolescents with I.D.D.M. *Diabetes Care, 10,* 752–758.

Hanson, C.L., Henggeler, S.W., Harris, M.A., Burghen, G.A. and Moore, M. (1989) Family system variables and the health status of adolescents with insulin-dependent diabetes mellitus. *Health Psychology, 8,* 239–253.

Hanson, C.L., Henggeler, S.W., Harris, M.A., Cigrang, J.A., Schinkel, A.M., Rodrigue, J.R. and Klesges, R.C. Contributions of sibling relations to the adoptation of youths with insulin-dependent diabetes mellitus. *Journal of Consulting and Clinical Psychology.*

Hanson, C.L., Henggeler, S.W., Rodrigue, J.R., Burghen, G.A. and Murphy, W.D. (1988) Father-absent adolescents with insulin-dependent diabetes mellitus: A population at risk? *Journal of Applied Developmental Psychology, 9,* 243–252.

Harder, C.F. and Bowditch, A. (1982) The impact of cystic fibrosis on siblings. *Children's Health Care, 14,* 141–145.

Hare, E.H., Lawrence, K.M., Payne, H. and Rawnsley, K. (1966) Spina bifida cystica and family stress. *British Medical Journal, 2,* 756–760.

Harter, S. (1985) *Teacher's Rating Scale of Child's Actual Behaviour*. Denver: University of Denver.

Harter, S. and Pike, R. (1984) The pictorial scale of perceived competence and social acceptance for young children. *Child Development, 55*, 1962–1982.

Hartup, W.W. (1983) Peer relations. In P.H. Mussen and E.M. Hetherington (eds.) *Handbook of Child Psychology, Vol. 4: Socialization, Personality and Social Development*. New York: Wiley, pp.103–196.

Harvey, D.H. and Greenway, A.P. (1984) The self-concept of physically handicapped children and their nonhandicapped siblings: An empirical investigation. *Journal of Child Psychology and Psychiatry, 25*, 273–284.

Hauenstein, E.J. (1987) *Families and Illness: Family Function and Adaptation in Families of Ill Children*. Charlottesville, VA: University of Virginia, Institute of Clinical Psychology.

Hauenstein, E.J. (1990) The experience of distress in parents of chronically ill children: Potential or likely outcome? *Journal of Clinical Child Psychology, 19*, 356–364.

Hauenstein, E.J., Marvin, R.S., Snyder, A.L. and Clarke, W.L. (1989) Stress in parents of children with diabetes mellitus. *Diabetes Care, 12*, 18–23.

Havermans, T. and Eiser, C. (1991) Locus of control and efficacy in healthy children and those with diabetes. *Psychology and Health, 5*, 297–306.

Havermans, T. and Eiser, C. (1991) Mothers' perceptions of parenting a child with spina bifida. *Child: Care, Health and Development, 17*, 259–273.

Haynes, R.B., Taylor, D.W. and Sackett, D.L. (1979) (eds.) *Compliance in Health Care*. Baltimore and London: John Hopkins University Press.

Heffron, W.A., Bommelaere, K. and Masters, R. (1976) Group discussions with parents of leukemia children. *Pediatrics, 52*, 831–840.

Hergenrather, J.R. and Rabinowitz, M. (1991) Age-related differences in the organization of children's knowledge of illness. *Developmental Psychology, 27*, 952–959.

Hibbard, J.H. and Pope, C.R. (1983) Gender roles, illness orientation, and use of medical services. *Social Science and Medicine, 17*, 129–137.

Hicks, R.A. and Hicks, M.J. (1991) Attitudes of major employers toward the employment of people with epilepsy: A 30-year study. *Epilepsia, 32*, 86–88.

Hill, J.P. (1987) Research on adolescents and their families: Past and prospect. In C.E. Irwin (ed.) *Adolescent Social Behaviour and Health*. San Francisco: Jossey-Bass. (pp.15–32).

Hill, R.A. (1988) Comment: Asthma in schools; *Respiratory Disease in Practice, 5*.

Hill, R.A., Standen, P.J. and Tattersfield, A.E. (1989) Asthma, wheezing, and school absence in primary schools. *Archives of Disease in Childhood, 64*, 246–251.

Hoare, P. (1984) Psychiatric disturbance in the families of epileptic children. *Developmental Medicine and Child Neurology, 26*, 14–19.

Hoare, P. and Kerley, S. (1991) Psychosocial adjustment of children with chronic epilepsy and their familes. *Developmental Medicine and Child Neurology, 33*, 201–215.

Hobfoll, S.E. (1986) (ed.) *Stress Social Support and Women*. Washington, D.C.: Hemisphere.

Hobfoll, S.E. (1991) Gender differences in stress reactions: Women filling the gaps. *Psychology and Health, 5*, 95–110.

Hobfoll, S.E. and Lerman, M. (1988) Personal relationships, personal attributes, and stress resistance: Mothers reactions to their child's illness. *American Journal of Community Psychology; 16*, 565–589.

Hobfoll, S.E. and Lerman, M. (1991) Predicting receipt of social support: A longitudinal study of parents' reactions to their child's illness. *Health Psychology, 8*, 61–77.

Hoffman, L.W. and Manis, G.B. (1978) Influences of children on marital interaction and parental satisfactions and dissatisfactions. In R.M. Lerner and G.B. Spanier (eds.) *Child Influences on Marital and Family Interaction: A Life-Span Perspective*. New York: Academic Press. pp.164–214.

Holden, A.E. and Barlow, D.H. (1986) Heart rate and heart rate variability recorded in vivro in agorophobics and nonphobics. *Behaviour Therapy, 17*, 26–42.

Holden, G.W. and Edwards, L.A. (1989) Parental attitudes toward child rearing: Instruments, issues and implications. *Psychological Bulletin, 106*, 29–58.

Holdsworth, L. and Whitmore, K. (1974) A study of children with epilepsy attending ordinary schools: I. Their seizure patterns, progress and behaviour in school. *Developmental Medicine and Child Neurology, 16*, 746–758.

Horowitz, M.J. and Kaltreider, N.B. (1980) Brief psychotherapy of stress response syndromes. In T. Karasu and L. Bellak (eds.) *Specialized Techniques in Individual Psychotherapy*. New York: Brunner/Mazel (pp.162–183).

Horwitz, W.A. and Kazak, A.E. (1990) Family adaptation to childhood cancer: Sibling and family system variables. *Journal of Clinical Child Psychology, 19*, 221–228.

Iles, P.J. (1974) Children with cancer: Healthy siblings' perception during the illness experience. *Cancer Nursing, 2*, 371–377.

Ilfield, F. (1976) Further validation of a Psychiatric Symptom Index in a normal population. *Psychological Reports, 39*, 1215–1228.

Ingersoll, G.M., Orr, D.P., Alison, J.H. and Golden, M.P. (1986) Cognitive maturity and self-management among adolescents with insulin-dependent diabetes mellitus. *Behavioural Pediatrics, 108*, 620–623.

Jacobsen, P.B., Manne, S.L., Gorfinkle, K., Schorr, O., Rapkin, B. and Redd, W.H. (1990) Analysis of child and parent behaviour during painful medical procedures. *Health Psychology, 9*, 559–576.

Jacobson, A., Barofsky, I., Cleary, P. and Rand, L. (1988) Reliability and validity of a diabetes quality-of-life measure for the diabetes control and complications trial (DCT) *Diabetes Care, 11*, 725–732.

Jacobson, A.M., Hauser, S.T., Wolfsdorf, Y.I., Hailihan, J., Milley, J.E., Herksowitz, R.D., Wertlieb, D. and Watt, E. (1987) Psychological predictions of compliance in children with recent onset of diabetes mellitus. *Journal of Pediatrics, 110*, 805–811.

Jay, S.M. and Elliott, C.H. (1984) Behavioural observation scales for measuring children's distress: The effects of increased methodological rigor. *Journal of Consulting and Clinical Psychology, 52,* 1106–1107.

Jay, S.M., Oxolins, M. and Elliot, C.H. (1983) Assessment of children's distress during painful medical procedures. *Health Psychology, 2,* 133–147.

Jenkins, J.M. and Smith, M.A. (1990) Factors protecting children living in disharmonious homes: Maternal reports. *Journal of the American Academy of Child and Adolescent Psychiatry, 29,* 60–69.

Jennings, K.D., Connors, R.E., Stegman, C.E., Sankaranayan, P. and Mendelsohn, S. (1985) Mastery motivation in young preschoolers: Effect of a physical handicap and implications for education and programming. *Journal of the Division for Early Childhood, 9,* 162–169.

Jessop, D.J., Reissman, C.K., and Stein, R.E.K. (1988) Chronic childhood illness and maternal mental health. *Journal of Developmental and Behavioural Pediatrics, 9,* 147–156.

Johnson, S.B. (1980) Psychosocial factors in juvenile diabetes: A review. *Journal of Behavioural Medicine, 3,* 95–116.

Johnson, S.B. (1988) Psychological aspects of childhood diabetes. *Journal of Child Psychology and Psychiatry, 29,* 729–739.

Johnson, S.B., Pollak, T., Silverstein, J.H., Rosenbloom, A.L., Spillar, R., McCallum, M. and Harkavy, J. (1982) Cognitive and behavioural knowledge about insulin-dependent diabetes among children and parents. *Pediatrics, 69,* 708–713.

Jones, O.H.M. (1980) Prelinguistic communication skills in Down's Syndrome and normal infants. In T. Field, S. Goldberg and D. Stern (eds.) *High Risk Infants and Children: Interactions with Adults and Peers.* New York: Academic Press.

Kagen-Goodhart, L. (1977) Re-entry: Living with childhood cancer. *American Journal of Orthopsychiatry, 47,* 651–658.

Kalnins, I.V. (1983) Cross-illness comparison of separation and divorce among parents having a child with a life-threatening illness. *Children's Health Care, 12,* 72–77.

Kalnins, I.V., Churchill, M.P. and Terry, G.E. (1980) Concurrent stresses in families with a leukemia child. *Journal of Pediatric Psychology, 5,* 81–92.

Kaplan, D.M., Grobstein, R. and Smith A. (1976) Predicting the impact of severe illness in families. *Health and Social Work, 13,* 72–82.

Katriel, T. and Philipsen, G. (1981) 'What we need is communication' as a cultural category in some American speech. *Communication Monographs, 48,* 301–318.

Katz, E.R., Kellerman, J. and Siegel, S.E. (1980) Behavioural distress in children with cancer undergoing medical procedures: Developmental considerations. *Journal of Consulting and Clinical Psychology, 48,* 356–365.

Kazak, A. and Meadows, A.T. (1988) Families of young adolescents who have survived cancer: Social-emotional adjustment, adaptability and social support. *Journal of Pediatric Psychology, 14,* 175–192.

Kazak, A., Reber, M. and Snitzer, L. (1988) Childhood chronic disease and family functioning: A study of phenylketonuria. *Pediatrics, 81,* 224–230.

Kazak, A.E. (1989) Families of chronically ill children: A systems and social-ecological model of adaptation and challenge. *Journal of Consulting and Clinical Psychology, 57,* 25–30.

⁕ Kazak, A.E. (1992) The social context of coping with childhood chronic illness: Family systems and social support. In A.M. La Greca, L.J. Siegel, J.L. Wallander and C.E. Walker (eds.) *Stress and Coping in Child Health.* New York: The Guilford Press. (pp.262–278).

Kazak, A.E. and Marvin, R.S. (1984) Differences, difficulties, and adaptation: Stress and social networks in families with a handicapped child. *Family Relations, 33,* 67–77.

Kazak, A.E. and Wilcox, B. (1984) The structure and function of social support networks in families with a handicapped child. *American Journal of Community Psychology, 12,* 645–661.

Kazak, A.E., Reber, M. and Carter, A. (1988) Structural and qualitative aspects of social networks in families with young chronically ill children. *Journal of Pediatric Psychology, 13,* 171–182.

Kendrick, C., Culling, J., Oakhill, T. and Mott, M. (1986) Children's understanding of their illness and its treatment within a paediatric oncology unit. *Association for Child Psychology and Psychiatry* (Newsletter) *8,* 16–20.

Kinrade, L.C. (1985) Preventive group intervention with siblings of oncology patients. *Childrens' Health Care, 14,* 110–113.

Kirk, C.R. and Savage, D.C.L. (1985) The diabetic with a diabetic parent. *Archives of Disease in Childhood, 60,* 572–586.

⟍ Kister, M.C. and Patterson, C.J. (1980) Childrens' conceptions of the causes of illness: understanding of contagion and use of immanent justice. *Child Development, 51,* 839–846.

Klein, S. and Simmons, R. (1979) Chronic disease and childhood development: Kidney disease and transplantation. In R. Simmons (ed.) *Research in Community and Mental Health,* Vol. 1. Greenwich, CT: JAI Press, p.3–20.

Klein, S.D. (1976) Measuring the outcome of the impact of chronic illness in childhood on the family. In G.D. Grave and I. Pless (eds.) *Chronic Childhood Illness: Assessment of Outcome.* Washington, D.C.: U.S. Department of Health, Education and Welfare.

Kochanska, G., Kuczynski, L. and Radke-Yarrow, M. (1989) Correspondence between mothers' self-reported and observed child-rearing practices. *Child Development, 60,* 56–63.

Koocher, G.P. (1986) Psychosocial issues during the acute treatment of pediatric cancer. *Cancer, 58,* 468–472.

Koocher, G.P. and O'Malley, J.E. (1981) (eds.) *The Damocles Syndrome: Psychological Consequences of Surviving Childhood Cancer.* New York: McGraw-Hill.

Korsch, B.M., Fine, R.N. and Negrette, V.F. (1978) Non-compliance in children with renal disease. *Pediatrics, 61,* 872–876.

Koski, M.L. (1969) The coping processes in childhood diabetes. *Acta Paediatric Scandinavica Suppl. 198,* 7–56.

Kovacs, M., Finkelstein, R., Feinberg, T.L., Crowse-Novak, M., Paulauskas, S. and Pollock, M. (1985) Initial psycholigical responses of parents to the diagnosis of insulin-dependent diabetes mellitus in their children. *Diabetes Care, 8,* 568–575.

Kovacs, M., Iyengar, S., Goldston, D., Stewart, J., Obrosky, S. and Marsh, J. (1990) Psychological functioning of children with insulin-dependent diabetes melliuts: A longitudinal study. *Journal of Pediatric Psychology, 15,* 619–632.

Kovaks, M., Kass, R.E., Schnell, T.M., Goldston, D. and Marsh, J. (1989) Family functioning and metabolic control of school-aged children with IDDM. *Diabetes Care, 12,* 409–414.

Krahn, G.L., Eisert, D. and Fifield, B. (1990) Obtaining parental perceptions of the quality of services for children with special health needs. *Journal of Pediatric Psychology, 15,* 761–774.

Kronenberger, W. and Thompson, R.J. (1990) Dimensions of family functioning in families with chronically ill children: A higher order factor analysis of the Family Environment Scale. *Journal of Clinical Child Psychology, 19,* 380–388.

Kubler-Ross, E. (1969) *On Death and Dying.* New York: MacMillan.

Kuczynski, L. and Kochanska, G. (1990) Development of children's non-compliance strategies from toddlerhood to age 5. *Developmental Psychology, 26,* 398–408.

Kupst, M.J. (1992) Long-term coping with acute lymphoblastic leukemia in childhood. In A.M. La Greca, L.J. Siegel, J.L. Wallander and C.E. Walker (eds.) *Stress and Coping in Child Health.* New York: Guildford Press. (pp.242–261).

Kupst, M.J. and Schulman, J.L. (1980) Family coping with leukemia in a child: Initial reactions. In J.L. Schulman and M.J. Kupst (eds.) *The Child with Cancer: Clinical Approaches to Psychosocial Care-Research in Psychosocial Aspects.* Springfield, IL: Charles C. Thomas (pp.111–128).

Kupst, M.J. and Schulman, J.L. (1988) Long-term coping with pediatric leukemia: A six-year follow-up study. *Journal of Pediatric Psychology, 13,* 7–22.

Kupst, M.J., Schulman, J.L., Honig, G., Maurer, H., Morgan, E. and Fochtman, D. (1982) Family coping with childhood leukemia: One year after diagnosis. *Journal of Pediatric Psychology, 7,* 157–174.

Kupst, M.J., Schulman, J.L., Maurer, H., Morgan, E., Honig, G. and Fochtman, D. (1984) Coping with pediatric leukemia: A two-year follow-up. *Journal of Pediatric Psychology, 9,* 149–163.

Kurdeck, L.A. (1981) An integrative perspective on children's divorce adjustment. *American Psychologist, 36,* 856–866.

La Greca, A.M. (1988) Adherence to prescribed medical regimens. In D. Routh (ed.) *Handbook of Pediatric Psychology.* New York: Guilford Press, pp.299–320.

La Greca, A.M. (1990a) Issues in adherence with pediatric regimens. *Journal of Pediatric Psychology, 15,* 423–436.

La Greca, A.M. (1990b) Social consequences of pediatric conditions: A fertile area for future investigation and intervention? *Journal of Pediatric Psychology, 15,* 285–307.

La Rossa, R. (1986) *Becoming a Parent.* Beverly Hills, CA: Sage.

Lancaster, S., Prior, M. and Adler, R. (1989) Child behaviour ratings: The influence of maternal characteristics and child temperament. *Journal of Child Psychology and Psychiatry, 30,* 137–150.

Langford, W.F. (1948) Physical illness and convalescence: Their meaning to the child. *Pediatrics, 33,* 242–250.

Lansdown, R., Atherton, D., Dale, A., Sproston, S. and Lloyd, J. (1986) Practical and psychological problems for parents of children with epidermolysis bullosa. *Child: Care, Health and Development, 12,* 251–256.

Lansky, S.B., Cairns, N.V. and Zwartjes, W. (1983) School attendance among children with cancer: A report from two centres. *Journal of Psychological Oncology, 1,* 75–82.

Lansky, S.B., Cairns, N.V., Hassanein, R., Mehr, J. and Lowman, J.T. (1978) Childhood cancer: Parental discord and divorce. *Pediatrics, 62,* 184–188.

Lansky, S.B., Lowman, J.T., Vats, T. and Gyulay, J.E. (1975) School phobia in children with malignant neoplasms. *American Journal of Diseases of Children, 129,* 42–46.

Larcombe, I.J., Walker, J., Charlton, A., Mellor, S., Morris-Jones, P. and Mott, M.G. (1990) Impact of childhood cancer on return to normal schooling. *British Medical Journal, 301,* 169–171.

· Lascari, A.D. and Stehbens, J.A. (1973) The reactions of families to childhood leukemia: An evaluation of a program of emotional management. *Clinical Pediatrics, 12,* 210–214.

Lauer, M., Mulhern, R., Wallskig, J. and Camitta, B. (1983) A comparison study of parental adaptation following a child's death at home or in the hospital. *Pediatrics, 71,* 107–111.

ι Lavigne, J. and Ryan, M. (1979) Psychological adjustments of siblings with chronic illness. *Pediatrics, 63,* 616–627.

· Lavigne, J.V., Irassman, H.S., Marr, T.J. and Chasnoff, I.J. (1982) Parental perceptions of the psychological adjustment of children with diabetes and their siblings. *Diabetes Care, 5,* 420–426.

Lavigne, J.V., Nolan, D. and McLone, D.G. (1988) Temperament, coping and psychological adjustment in young children with myelomeningocele. *Journal of Pediatric Psychology, 13,* 363–378.

Lazarus, R.S. and Folkman, S. (1984) *Stress, Appraisal and Coping.* New York: Springer.

Leaverton, D.R. (1979) The child with diabetes mellitus. In J.D. Call, J.D. Nosphpize, R.I. Cohen and I. Berlin (eds.) *Basic Handbook of Child Psychiatry,* Vol. 1, New York: Basic Books.

Lebow, J. (1983) Similarities and differences between mental health and health care evaluation studies assessing consumer satisfaction. *Evaluation and Program Planning, 6,* 237–245.

Lemanek, K. (1991) Adherence issues in the medical management of asthma. *Journal of Pediatric Psychology, 15,* 437–458.

Lenarsky, C. and Feig, S. (1983) Bone marrow transplantation for children with cancer. *Pediatric Annals, 12,* 428–436.

Lepore, S.J. and Kliewer, W. (1989) Monitoring and blunting: Validation of a coping measure for children. Paper presented at American Psychological Association Convention, New Orleans.

Lesko, L.M., Dermatis, H., Penman, D. and Holland, J.C. (1989) Patients', parents' and oncologists' perceptions of informed consent for bone marrow transplantation. *Medical and Pediatric Oncology, 17*, 181–187.

Lester, B. and Zeskind, P.S. (1979) The organization and assessment of crying in the infant at risk. In T. Field, A. Sostek, S. Goldberg and H. Shuman (eds.) *Infants Born at Risk.* New York: SP Medical and Scientific Books.

Levenson, P.M. and Cooper, M.A. (1984) School health education for the chronically impaired individual. *Journal of School Health, 54*, 466–449.

Levenson, P.M., Copeland, D.R., Morrow, J.R., Pfefferbaum, B. and Silberberg, Y. (1983) Disparities in disease-related perceptions of adolescent cancer patients and their parents. *Journal of Pediatric Psychology, 8*, 33–45.

Levy, D.M. (1943) *Maternal Overprotection.* New York: Columbia University Press.

Lewis, R.A. and Spanier, G. (1979) Theorizing about the quality and the stability of marriage. In W.R. Burr, R. Hill, F.I. Nye and I.L. Reiss (eds.) *Contemporary Theories about the Family* Vol. 1. pp.268–294. New York: Free Press.

Li, F.P. and Stone, R. (1976) Survivors of cancer in childhood. *Annals of Internal Medicine, 84*, 551–553.

Linde, L.M., Rosof, B. and Dunn, O.J. (1970) Longitudinal studies of intellectual and behavioural development in children with congenital heart disease. *Acta Paediatrica Scandinavica, 59*, 169–176.

Linde, L.M., Rosof, B., Dunn, O.J. and Robb, E. (1966) Attitudinal factors in congenital heart disease. *Pediatrics, 38*, 92–101.

Lineberger, H.O. (1981) Social characteristics of a hemophilia clinic population. *General Hospital Psychiatry, 3*, 157–163.

Liptak, G.S. (1987) Spina bifida. In R.A. Hoekelman, S. Blatman, S.B. Friedman, N.M. Nelson and H.M. Seidel (eds.) *Primary Pediatric Care.* St. Louis: C.V. Mosby (pp.1487–1492).

Litt, I.F. and Cuskey, W.R. (1980) Compliance with medical regimens during adolescence. *Pediatric Clinics of North America, 27*, 3–15.

Lobato, D., Faust, D. and Spirito, A. (1988). Examining the effects of chronic disease and disability on children's sibling relationships. *Journal of Pediatric Psychology, 13*, 389–408.

Loyd, B.H. and Abidin, R.A. (1985) Revision of the Parenting Stress Index. *Journal of Pediatric Psychology, 10*, 169–178.

Madan-Swain, A. and Brown, R.T. (1991) Cognitive and psychosocial sequelae for children with acute lymphocytic leukemia and their families. *Clinical Psychology Review, 11*, 267–293.

Malpas, J.S. (1988) The consequences of cure. *Clinical Radiology, 39*, 166–172.

Markova, I., MacDonald, K. and Forbes, C. (1980) Integration of haemophilic boys into normal schools. *Child: Care, Health and Development, 6*, 101–109.

Marteau, T.M. and Baum, J.D. (1984) Doctors' views on diabetes. *Archives of Disease in Childhood, 59*, 566–570.

Martin, P. (1975) Marital breakdown in families of patients with spina bifida cystica. *Developmental Medicine and Child Neurology, 17,* 757–764.

Matas, L., Arend, R.A., Sroufe, L.A. (1978) Continuity and adaptation in the second year: The relationship between quality of attachment and later competence. *Child Development, 49,* 549–556.

McCarthy, M. (1975) The care of childhood leukemia in general practice. *Journal of the Royal College of General Practitioners, 25,* 286–292.

McCauley, E., Kay, T., Ito, J. and Treder, R. (1987) The Turner syndrome: Cognitive deficits, effective discrimination, and behaviour problems. *Child Development, 58,* 464–474.

McCrae, R.R. (1984) Situational determinants of coping responses: Loss, threat and challenge. *Journal of Personality and Social Psychology, 46,* 919–928.

McCubbin, H.I., Cauble, A.E. and Patterson, J.M. (1982) (eds.) *Family Stress, Coping and Social Support.* Springfield, IL: Charles C. Thomas.

McCubbin, H.I., McCubbin, M.A., Patterson, J.M., Cauble, A.E., Wilson, L.R. and Warwick, W. (1983) CHIP – Coping Health Inventory for Parents: An assessment of parental coping patterns in the care of the chronically ill child. *Journal of Marriage and the Family,* May, 359–370.

McHale, S. and Gamble, W. (1987) Relationship between handicapped children and their non-handicapped siblings and peers. In J. Garbarino, T. Brookhauser and K. Authier (eds.) *Special Children – Special Risks: The Maltreatment of Handicapped Children.* New York: Aldine.

McHale, S.M., Bartko, W., Crouter, A.C. and Perry-Jenkins, M. (1990) Children's housework and psychosocial functioning: The mediating effects of parents' sex-role behaviours and attitudes. *Child Development, 61,* 1413–1426.

McKeever, P. (1983) Siblings of chronically ill children: A literature review with implications for research and practice. *American Journal of Orthopsychiatry, 53,* 209–218.

McKeever, P.T. (1981) Fathering the chronically ill child. *American Journal of Maternal Child Nursing, 6,* 124–128.

McNabb, W.L., Wilson-Pessano, S.R. and Jacobs, A.M. (1986) Critical self-management competencies for children with asthma. *Journal of Pediatric Psychology, 11,* 103–118.

Melamed, B. (1992) Family factors predicting children's reactions to anesthesia induction. In A.M., LaGreca, C.J., Siegel, J.L. Wallander and C.E. Walker (eds.) *Stress and Coping in Child Health.* New York: Guilford Press, pp.140–156.

Melamed, B.G. and Bush, J. (1986) Maternal–child influences during medical procedures. In S. Allerbach and S. Stolberg (eds.) *Crisis Intervention with Children and Families.* Washington, D.C.: Hemishpere.

Melamed, B.G. and Siegel, L. (1975) Reduction of anxiety in children facing hospitalization and surgery by use of filmed modeling. *Journal of Consulting and Clinical Psychology, 43,* 511–521.

Melamed, B.G. and Siegel, L.J. (1980) *Behavioural Medicine: Practical Applications in Health-Care.* New York: Springer.

Melamed, B.G., Dearborn, M. and Hermecz, D.A. (1983) Necessary conditions for surgery preparation: Age and previous experience. *Psychosomatic Medicine, 45,* 517–525.

Menke, E.M. (1987) The impact of a child's illness on school-aged siblings. *Children's Health Care, 15,* 132–140.

Meyerowitz, J.H. and Kaplan, H.B. (1967) Familial response to stress: The case of cystic fibrosis. *Social Science and Medicine, I,* 249–266.

Milberg, W., Hebben, N. and Kaplan, E. (1986) The Boston approach to neuropsychological assessment. In K. Adams and I. Grant (eds.) *Neuropsychological Assessment of Neuropsychiatric Disorders* (pp.65–86) New York: Oxford University Press.

Miller, J.J., Spitz, P.W., Simpson, V. and Williams, G.F. (1982) The social function of young adults who had arthritis in childhood. *Journal of Pediatrics, 100,* 378–382.

Miller, S. (1980) When is a little information a dangerous thing? Coping with stressful life events by monitoring vs blunting. In S. Levine and H. Ursin (eds.) *Coping and Health,* New York: Plenum (pp.145–169).

Miller, S. (1987) Monitoring and blunting: Validation of a questionnaire to assess styles of information seeking under threat. *Journal of Personality and Social Psychology, 52,* 345–353.

Millstein, S.G., Adler, N.E. and Irwin, C.E. (1981) Conceptions of illness in young adolescents. *Pediatrics, 68,* 834–839.

Moos, R. (1974) *The Family Environment Scale.* Palo Alto, CA: Consulting Psychologists Press.

Moos, R.G. and Moos, B.S. (1981) *Family Environment Scale.* Palo Alto, CA: Consulting Psychologists Press.

Moss, H.A., Nanis, E.D. and Poplack, D.G. (1981) The effects of prophylactic treatment of the central nervous system on the intellectual functioning of children with acute lymphocytic leukemia. *American Journal of Medicine, 1981, 71,* 47–52.

Mulhern, R.K., Crisco, J.J. and Camitta, B.M. (1981) Patterns of communication among pediatric patients with leukemia, parents and physicians; prognostic disagreements and misunderstanding. *Journal of Pediatrics, 99,* 480–483.

Mulhern, R.K., Wasserman, A.L., Friedman, A.G. and Fairclough, D. (1989) Social competence and behavioural adjustment of children who are long-term survivors of cancer. *Pediatrics, 83,* 18–25.

Murphy, L.B. and Moriarty, A.E. (1976) *Vulnerability, Coping and Growth.* New Haven, CT: Yale University Press.

Nagy, S. and Ungerer, J. (1990) The adaptation of mothers and fathers to children with cystic fibrosis: A comparison. *Children's Health Care, 19,* 147–154.

Nazarian, L.R., Maiman, L.A. and Bocker, M.H. (1989) Recruitment of a large community of pediatricians in a collaborative research project. *Clinical Pediatrics, 28,* 210–213.

Nelson, K. (1986) (ed.) *Event Knowledge: Structure and Function in Development.* New Jersey: Lawrence Erlbaum.

Nevin, R.S., McCubbin, H.I. Birkebak, R.C. (1983) Assessment promotion of family coping with stressors in disability. *Pediatric Social Work, 3,* 23–30.

Nocon, A. (1991) Social and emotional impact of childhood asthma. *Archives of Disease in Childhood,* 459–460.

Nolan, T., Desmond, K., Herlich, R. and Hardy, S. (1986) Knowledge of cystic fibrosis in patients and their parents. *Pediatrics, 77,* 229–235.

‹ Noll, R.B., LeRoy, S., Bukowski, W.M. Rogosch, F.A. and Kulkarni, R. (1991) Peer relationships and adjustment in children with cancer. *Journal of Pediatric Psychology, 16,* 307–326.

Olson, D.H., Bell, R. and Portner, J. (1982) *FACES II.* St Paul MN: Family Social Science, University of Minnesota.

Olson, D.H., Russell, C.S. and Sprenkle, D.H. (1983) Model of marital and family systems. *Family Process, 22,* 69–83.

Olson, R.A., Holden, E.W., Friedman, A., Faust, J., Kenning, M. and Mason, P.J. (1988) Psychological consultation in a children's hospital: An evaluation of services. *Journal of Pediatric Psychology, 18,* 479–492.

Osborne, R.B., Hatcher, J.W. and Richtsmeier, A.J. (1989) The role of social modeling in unexplained pediatric pain. *Journal of Pediatric Psychology, 14,* 43–62.

Palfrey, J., Levy, J.C. and Gilbert, K.L. (1980) Use of primary care facilities by patients attending specialty clinics. *Pediatrics, 65,* 567–572.

Pantell, R.H., Stewart, T.J., Dias, J.K., Wells, P. and Ross, A.W. (1982) Physician communication with children and parents. *Pediatrics, 70,* 396–402.

Park, K.A. and Waters, E. (1989) Security of attachment and preschool friendships. *Child Development, 60,* 1076–1081.

Parke, R.D. (1979) Perspectives on father-infant interaction. In J. Osofsky (ed.), *Handbook of Infant Development,* New York: Wiley.

Parmalee, A.H. (1986) Children's illnesses: Their beneficial effects on behavioural development. *Child Development, 57,* 1–10.

Partridge, J.W., Garner, A.M., Thompson, C.W. and Cherry, T. (1972) Attitudes of adolescents toward their diabetes. *American Journal of Diseases of Children, 124,* 226–229.

Pasley, K. and Gecas, V. (1984) Stresses and satisfactions of the parental role. *Personal and Guidance Journal, 2,* 400–404.

Pearlman, D.S. (1984) Bronchial asthma: A perspective from childhood to adulthood. *American Journal of Diseases of Children, 138,* 459–466.

⌀ Peck, B. (1979) Effects of childhood cancer on long-term survivors and their families. *British Medical Journal, 1,* 1327–1329.

Peckham, V.C., Meadows, A.T., Bartel, N. and Marrero, O. (1988) Educational late effects in long-term survivors of childhood acute lymphocytic leukemia. *Pediatrics, 81,* 127–133.

Pederson, D., Evans, B., Chance, G., Bento, A. and Fox, A. (1988) Predictors of one-year developmental status in low birth weight infants. *Developmental and Behavioural Pediatrics, 9,* 287–292.

Perrin, E.C. and Gerrity, P.S. (1981) There's a demon in your belly: Children's understanding of illness. *Pediatrics*, 841–849.

Perrin, E.C., and Gerrity, B.S. (1984) Development of children with a chronic illness. *Pediatric Clinics of North America, 31*, 1–17.

Perrin, E.C., Sayer, A.G. and Willett, J.B. (1991) Sticks and stones may break my bones... Reasoning about illness causality and body functioning in children who have a chronic illness. *Pediatrics, 88*, 608–619.

Perrin, E.C., Stein, R.E.K. and Drotar, D. (1991) Cautions in using the Child Behaviour Checklist: Observations based on research about children with a chronic illness. *Journal of Pediatric Psychology, 16* 411–422.

Perrin, E.C., West, P.D., and Culley, B.S. (1989) Is my child normal yet? Correlates of vulnerability. *Pediatrics, 83*, 355–363.

Perrin, J.M. and MacLean, E.W. (1987) Education and stress management in childhood chronic illness. Final report to Williamson T. Grant Foundation, Grant No. 82–0836–00.

Perrin, J.M., MacLean, W.E. and Perrin, E.C. (1989) Parental perceptions of health status and psychologia adjustment of children with asthma. *Pediatrics, 83*, 26–30.

Peterson, L. and Mori, L. (1988) Preparation for hospitalization. In D. Routh (ed.) *Handbook of Pediatric Psychology*. New York: Guilford Press, pp.460–491.

Peterson, L. and Shigetomi, C. (1981) The use of coping techniques to minimize anxiety in hospitalised children. *Behaviour Therapy, 12*, 1–14.

Peterson, L. and Toler, S.M. (1986) An information seeking disposition in child surgery patients. *Health Psychology, 5*, 343–358.

Peterson, L., Harbeck, C., Farmer, J. and Zink, M. (1991) Developmental contributions to the assessment of children's pain: Conceptual and Methodological implications. In J.P. Bush and S.W. Harkins (eds.) *Children in Pain: Clinical and Research Issues from a Developmental Perspective*. New York: Springer-Verlag. (pp.33–58).

Pfefferbaum, B. and Levenson, P.M. (1982) Adolescent cancer patients and physician responses to a questionnaire on patient concerns. *American Journal of Psychiatry, 139*, 348–351.

Phipps, S. and DeCuir-Whalley, S. (1990) Adherence issues in pediatric bone-marrow transplantation. *Journal of Pediatric Psychology, 15*, 459–475.

Phipps, S. and Drotar, D. (1990) Determinants of parenting stress in home aphea monitoring. *Journal of Pediatric Psychology, 15*, 385–400.

Piaget, J. (1929) *The Child's Conception of the World*. New York: Harcourt Brace Jovanovich.

Piaget, J. (1952) *The Origins of Intelligence in Children*. New York: International Universities Press.

Pinelli, J.M. (1981) A comparison of mothers' concerns regarding the care-taking tasks of newborns with congenital heart disease before and after assuming their care. *Journal of Advanced Nursing, 6*, 261–270.

Pinto, R.P. and Hollandsworth, J.G. (1984) Preparing parents of pediatric surgical patients using a videotape model. Paper presented at the meeting of the Society of behavioural Medicine, Philadelphia.

Pless, I.B. (1984) Clinical assessment: Physical and psychological functioning. *Pediatric Clinics of North America, 31,* 33–46.

Pless, I.B. and Pinkerton, P. (1975) *Chronic Childhood Disorder: Promoting Patterns of Adjustment.* London: Henry Kimpton.

Plomin, R. and Daniels, D. (1987) Why are children in the same family so different from one another? *Behavioural and Brain Sciences, 10,* 1–22.

Plunkett, J., Meisles, S. and Stiefel, G. (1986) Patterns of attachment among preterm infants of varying biological risk. *Journal of the American Academy of Child Psychiatry, 25,* 794–798.

Poplack, D.G. (1988) Acute lymphoblastic leukemia. In P.A. Pizzo and D.G. Poplack (eds.) *Principles and Practice of Pediatric Oncology,* (pp.323–366). Philadelphia, PA: Lippincott.

Pot-Mees, C. (1989) *The Psychosocial Effects of Bone Marrow Transplantation in Children.* Delft, The Netherlands: Eburon.

Potter, P.C. and Roberts, M.C. (1984) Children's perceptions of chronic illness: The roles of disease symptoms, cognitive development and information. *Journal of Pediatric Psychology, 9,* 13–28.

Powazek, M., Schijring, J., Goff, J.R., Paulson, M.A. and Stegner, S. (1980) Psychosocial ramifications of childhood leukemia: One year post diagnosis. In J.L. Schulman and M.J. Kupst (eds.) *The Child with Cancer.* Springfield, IC: Charles C. Thomas pp.143–155.

Powell, T.H. and Ogle, P.A. (1985) *Brothers and Sisters – A Special Part of Exceptional Families.* Baltimore: Paul H. Brookes.

Quittner, A.L. (1992) Re-examining research on stress and social support: The importance of contextual factors. In A.M., La Greca, L.J., Siegel, J.L. Wallander and C.E. Walker (eds.) *Stress and Coping in Child Health.* New York: Guilford Press, (pp.85–117).

Reed, C.E. and Townley, R.G. (1983) Asthma: Classification and pathogenesis. In E., Middleton, Jnr., C.E. Reed and E.F. Ellis (eds.) *Allergy: Principles and Practice* (2nd ed.) St. Louis: Mosby.

Reissland, N. (1985) The development of concepts of simultaneity in children's understanding of emotion. *Journal of Child Psychology and Psychiatry, 26,* 5, 811–824.

Reynolds, J.M., Garralda, M.E., Postlethwaite, R.J. and Goh, D. (1988) Changes in psychosocial adjustment after renal transplantation. *Archives of Disease in Childhood, 66,* 508–513.

Richman, N. (1977) Behaviour problems in pre-school children: Family and social factors. *British Journal of Psychiatry, 131,* 523–527.

Richman, N., Stevenson, J. and Graham, P.J. (1982) *Pre-School to School: A Behavioural Study.* London: Academic Press.

Roberts, M.C. (1986) *Pediatric psychology: Psychological Interventions and Strategies for Pediatric Problems.* New York: Pergamon.

Robinson, N., Bush, L., Protopapa, L.E. and Yateman, N.A. (1989b) Employers' attitudes to diabetes. *Diabetic Medicine, 6*, 692–697.

Robinson, N., Yateman, N.A., Protopapa, L.E. and Bush, L. (1989a) Unemployment and diabetes. *Diabetic Medicine, 6*, 797–803.

Roghmann, K. and Haggerty, R. (1972) Family stress and the use of health services. *International Journal of Epidemiology, 1*, 279–286.

Rollins, B.C. and Feldman, H. (1970) Marital satisfaction over the family life-cycle. *Journal of Marriage and the Family, 32*, 20–28.

Rothbaum, F., Weisz, J.R. and Snyder, S.S. (1982) Changing the world and changing the self: A two-process model of perceived control. *Journal of Personality and Social Psychology, 42*, 5–37.

Rovet, J.F., Ehrlich, R.M. and Hoppe, M. (1987) Intellectual deficits associated with early onset of insulin-dependent diabetes mellitus in children. *Diabetes Care, 10*, 510–515.

Rutter, M. (1979) Protective factors in children's responses to stress and disadvantage. In M.W. Kent and J. Rolf (eds.) *Social Competence in Children.* Hanover: N.H. University Press of New England, Vol. 3.

Rutter, M. (1981) Stress, coping and development: Some issues and some questions. *Journal of Child Psychology and Psychiatry, 22*, 323–356.

Rutter, M., Tizard, J. and Whitmore, K. (1970) *Education, Health and Behaviour.* New York: Wiley and Sons.

Ryan, C., Vega, A. and Drash, A. (1985) Cognitive deficits in adolescents who developed diabetes early in life. *Pediatrics, 75*, 921–927.

Ryan, C.M. (1990) Neuro-psychological consequences and correlates of diabetes in childhood. In C.S. Holmes (ed.) *Neuropsychological and behavioural aspects of diabetes.* New York: Springer-Verlag, (pp.58–84).

Saarni, C. and Harris, P.L. (eds.) (1989) *Children's understanding of emotion.* UK: Cambridge University Press.

Sabbeth, B. and Stein, R.E.K. (1990) Mental health referral: A weak link in comprehensive care of children with chronic physical illness. *Developmental and Behavioural Pediatrics, 11*, 73–78.

Sabbeth, B.F. and Leventhal, J.M. (1984) Marital adjustment to chronic childhood illness: A critique of the literature. *Pediatrics, 73*, 762–768.

Sachs, M.B. (1980) Helping the child with cancer go back to school. *Journal of School Health, August*, 328–331.

Saille, H., Burgmeier, R. and Schmidt, L.R. (1988) A meta-analysis of studies on psychological preparation of children facing medical procedures. *Psychology and Health, 2*, 107–132.

Salmi, J., Huuponen, T. and Oksa, H., Oksala, A., Koivula, J. and Raita, S. (1986) Metabolic control in adolescent insulin-dependent diabetics referred from pediatric to adult clinic. *Annals of Clinical Research, 18*, 84–87.

Sameroff, A.J. and Chandler, M.J. (1975) Reproductive risk and the continuum of caretaking casualty. In F.D. Horwitz (ed.) *Review of Child Development Research.* Chicago, IL: University of Chicago Press. (pp.187–243).

Sandberg, D.E., Meyer-Bahlber, H. and Yager, T.J. (1991) The Child Behaviour Checklist. Nonclinical standardized samples: Should they be utilized as norms? *Journal of the American Academy of Child and Adolescent Psychiatry, 30,* 124–134.

Sands, H. (1982) *Epilepsy: A Handbook for the Mental Health Professional.* Brunner/Mazel Publishers.

Sanger, M.S., Copeland, D.R. and Davidson, E.R. (1991) Psychosocial adjustment among pediatric cancer patients: A multidimensional assessment. *Journal of Pediatric Psychology, 16,* 463–474.

Sargent, J., Rossman, B., Baker, L., Nogiuiera, J. and Stanley, C. (1985) Family interaction and diabetic control: A prospective study. *Diabetes, 34,* (Suppl. 1), 77A.

Schacter, S., Shore, E., Feldman-Rotman, S., Marquis, R. and Campbell, S. (1976) Sibling deidentification. *Developmental Psychology, 12,* 412–427.

Schecter, N.L., Bernstein, B. Beck, A., Hart, L. and Scherzer, L. (1991) Individual differences in children's response to pain: Role of temperament and parental characteristics. *Pediatrics, 87,* 171–177.

Schidlow, D.V. and Fiel, S.B. (1990) Life beyond pediatrics: Transition of chronically ill adolescents from pediatric to adult health care systems. *Medical Clinics of North America, 74,* 1113–1120.

Schlieper, A., Alcock, D., Beaudry, P., Feldman, W., and Leikin, L. (1991) Effects of therapeutic plasma concentrations of theophylline on behaviour, cognitive processing, and affect in children with asthma. *Journal of Pediatrics, 118,* 449–455.

Schlosser, M. and Havermans, G. (1992) A self efficacy scale for children and adolescents with asthma: Construction and validation. *Journal of Asthma, 29,* 99–108.

Schwachman, H. and Kulczycki, L.L. (1985) Long-term study of 105 patients with cystic fibrosis: Studies made over a 5 to 14 year period. *American Journal of Diseases of Childhood, 96,* 6–15.

Seagull, E.A. and Somers, S. (1991) Autonomy expectations in families with chronically ill and healthy adolescents. Paper presented at the Third Florida Conference on Child Health Psychology, Gainesville, Florida, April 1991.

Shaw, E.G. and Routh, D.K. (1982) Effect of mother presence on children's reaction to aversive procedures. *Journal of Pediatric Psychology, 7,* 33–42.

Shouval, R., Ber, R. and Galatzer, A. (1982) Family social climate and the length, status and social adaptation of diabetic youth. In Z. Laron (ed.), *Psychological Aspects of Diabetes in Children and Adolescents.* Basel: Karger.

Siegel, L., Saigal, S., Rosenbaum, P., Morton, R., Young, A., Berenbaum, S. and Stoskopf, B. (1983) Predictors of development in preterm and full-term infants: A model for detecting the 'at-risk' child. *Journal of Pediatric Psychology, 7,* 135–148.

Siegel, S.E. (1980) The current outlook for childhood cancer: The medical background. In J. Kellerman (ed.) *Psychological Aspects of Childhood Cancer.* Springfield, IL: Charles Thomas.

Silbert, A.R., Newburger, J.W. and Fyler, D.C. (1982) Marital instability and congenital heart disease. *Pediatrics, 69,* 747–750.

Sillars, A., Pike, G.R., Jones, T.J. and Murphy, M.A.C. (1984) Communication and understanding in marriage. *Human Communication Research, 10,* 317–350.

Sillars, A.L., Weisberg, J., Burgraff, C.S. and Wilson, E.A. (1987) Content themes in marital conversations. *Human Communication Research, 13,* 495–528.

Simmons, R. and Blyth, D. (1987) *Moving into Adolescence: The Impact of Pubertal Change and School Context.* New York: Aldine de Grayter.

Skipper, J.K. Jnr., Leonard, R.L. and Rhymes, J. (1968) Child hospitalization and social interaction: An experimental study of mother's feelings of stress, adaptation and satisfacion. *Medical Care, 6,* 496–506.

Slavin, L.A., O'Malley, J.E., Koocher, G. and Foster, D.J. (1982) Communication of the cancer diagnosis to pediatric patients: Impact on long-term adjustment. *American Journal of Psychiatry, 139*(2), 179–183.

Small, S.E., Cornelius, S. and Eastman, G. (1983) Parenting adolescent children: A period of adult storm and stress? Paper presented at the annual meeting of the American Psychological Association, Montreal.

Smith, S.D., Rosen, D., Trueworthy, R.C. and Lowman, J.T. (1979) A reliable method for evaluating drug compliance in children with cancer. *Cancer, 43,* 169–173.

Snyder, D.K. and Regts, J.M. (1982) Factor scales for assessing marital disharming and disaffection. *Journal of Consulting and Clinical Psychology, 50,* 736–743.

Sourkes, B.M. (1987) Siblings of the child with a life-threatening illness. *Journal of Children in Contemporary Society, 19,* 159–184.

Spanier, G.B. (1976) Measuring dyadic adjustment: New scale for assessing the quality of marriage and similar dyads. *Journal of Marriage and the Family, 38,* 15–28.

Speltz, M.L., Armsden, G.C. and Clarren, S.S. (1990) Effects of craniofacial birth defects on maternal functioning postinfancy. *Journal of Pediatric Psychology, 15,* 177–196.

Spielberger, C.D. (1973) *Manual for the State-Trait Anxiety Inventory for Children.* Palo Alto, CA: Consulting Psychologists Press.

Spinetta, J.J. (1981) Adjustment and adaptation in children with cancer. In J.J. Spinetta and P. Spinetta (eds.) *Living with Childhood Cancer.* St Louis: Mosby.

Spirito, A., Stark, L.J. and Tyc, V. (1989) Common coping strategies employed by children with chronic illness. *Newsletter of the Society of Pediatric Psychology, 13,* 3–8.

Spirito, A., Stark, L.J., Williams, C., Stamoulis, D. and Axelson, D. (1988 April) Coping strategies utilized by referred and nonreferred pediatric patients and a healthy control group. Poster presented at the annual meeting of the Society of Behavioural Medicine, Boston.

Stark, L.J., Spirito, A. and Tyc, V. (1991) Coping strategies utilized by chronically ill and acutely ill hospitalized children. Manuscript submitted for publication, Rhode Island Hospital.

Stehbens, J.A. and Lascari, A.D. (1974) Psychological follow-up of families with childhood leukemia. *Journal of Clinical Psychology, 30,* 394–397.

Stein, R.E.K. and Jessop, D.J. (1982) A noncategorical approach to chronic childhood illness. *Public Health Reports, 97* 354–362.

Stein, R.E.K. and Jessop, D.J. (1984) Psychological adjustment among children with chronic conditions. *Pediatrics, 73,* 169–174.

Stein, R.E.K., Jessop, D.J. and Reissman, C.K. (1983) Health care services received by children with chronic illness. *American Journal of Diseases of Childhood, 137,* 225–230

Steinberg, L. (1985) *Adolescence.* New York: Random House.

Steinhauer, P. Mushin, D. and Rae-Grant, Q. (1983) Psychological aspects of chronic illness. In Steinhauer, P. and Rae-Grant, Q. (eds.) *Psychological Problems of the Child in his Family.* New York: Basic Books.

Stern, M. and Arenson, E. (1989) Childhood cancer stereotype: Impact on adult perceptions of children. *Journal of Pediatric Psychology, 14,* 593–606.

Stewart, D.A., Stein, A., Forrest, G.C. and Clark, D.M. (1992) Psychosocial adjustment in siblings of children with chronic life-threatening illness: A research note. *Journal of Child Psychology and Psychiatry, 33,* 779–784.

Stillar, C.A. and Draper, G.J. (1989) Treatment centre size, entry to trials, and survival in acute lymphoblastic leukemia. *Archives of Disease in Childhood, 64,* 657–661.

Strickland, D.E. and Pittman, D.J. (1984) Social learning and teenage alchohol use: interpersonal and observational influences within the social-cultural environment. *Journal of Drug Issues, 14,* 137–150.

Tattersall, R.B. and Jackson, J.G.L. (1982) Social and emotional complications of diabetes. In H. Keen and J. Jarrett (eds.) *Complications of Diabetes.* London: Ed. Arnold.

Tavormina, J.B., Kastner, L.S., Slater, P.M. and Watt, S.L. (1976) Chronically sick children: A psychological and emotionally deviant population. *Journal of Abnormal Child Psychology, 4,* 99–110.

Taylor, M.R.H. and O'Connor, P. (1989) Resident parents and shorter hospital stay. *Archives of Disease in Psychology, 64,* 274–276.

Tebbi, C.K. Koren, B.G. (1983) A specialized unit for adolescent oncology patients. Is it worth it? *Journal of Medicine, 14,* 161–184.

Tebbi, C.K., Cummings, K.M., Zevon, M.A., Smith, L., Richards, M. and Mallin, J. (1986) Compliance of pediatric and adolescent cancer patients. *Cancer, 58,* 1179–1184.

Tebbi, C.K., Richards, M.E., Cummings, K.M., Zevon, M.A. and Mallon, J.C. (1988) The role of parent-adolescent concordance in compliance with cancer chemotherapy. *Adolescence, 91,* 599–611.

Teta, M.J., Del Po, M.C., Kasl, S.V., Meigs, J.W., Myers, M.H. and Mulvihill, J.J. (1986) Psychosocial consequences of childhood and adolescent cancer survival. *Journal of Chronic Disease, 39,* 751–759.

Tew, B. (1977) Spina Bifida children's scores on the Wechsler Intelligence Scale for Children. *Perceptual and Motor Skills, 44,* 381–382.

Tew, B. and Laurence, K.M. (1973) Mothers, brothers and sisters of patients with spina bifida. *Developmental Medicine and Child Neurology, 15,* 69–76.

Tew, B., Payne, H. and Lawrence, V.M. (1974) 'Must a family with a handicapped child be a handicapped family?' *Developmental Medicine and Child Neurology, 16,* (Suppl. 32) 95–98.

Thoits, P.A. (1987) Gender and marital status differences in control and distress: Common Stress vs. unique stress explanations. *Journal of Health and Social behaviour, 28,* 7–22.

Tiller, J.W., Ekert, H. and Rickards, W.S. (1977) Family reactions in childhood acute lymphoblastic leukemia in remision. *Australian Pediatric Journal, 13,* 176–181.

Trause, M.A. and Kramer, L.I. (1983) The effects of premature birth on parents and their relationship. *Developmental Medicine and Child Neurology, 25,* 459–465.

Travis, G. (1978) *Chronic Illness in Childhood: Its Impact on Child and Family.* Stanford, CA: Stanford University Press.

Treffers, P.D.A., Goedhart, A.W., Waltz, J.W. and Kouldijs, P. (1990) The systematic collection of patient data in a centre for child and adolescent psychiatry. *British Journal of Psychiatry, 157,* 744–748.

Treiber, F.A., Schramm, L. and Mabe, P.A. (1986) Children's knowledge and concerns toward a peer with cancer: A workshop intervention approach. *Child Psychiatry and Human Development, 16,* 249–260.

Tritt, S.G. and Esses, L.M. (1988) Psychosocial adaptation of siblings of children with chronic medical illnesses. *American Journal of Orthopsychiatry, 58,* 211–220.

Tropauer, A., Franz, M.N. and Dilgard, V.W. (1970) Psychological aspects of the care of children with cystic fibrosis. *American Journal of Diseases of Children, 119,* 424–432.

Turk, J. (1964) Impact of cystic fibrosis on family functioning. *Pediatrics, 34,* 67–71.

Ungerer, J., Horgan, G., Chaitow, J. and Champion, G.B. (1988) Psychosocial functioning in children and young adults with juvenile arthritis. *Journal of Pediatrics, 81,* 195–202.

van der Veen, F. and Olson, R.E. (1983) *Manual and Handbook for the Family Concept Assessment Method.* California: Encinitas.

van der Veer, A.H. (1949) The psychopathology of physical illness and hospital residence. *Quarterly Journal of Child Behaviour, 1,* 55–71.

Vance, J.C., Fazan, C.E., Satterwhite, B. and Pless, I.B. Effects of nephrotic syndrome on the family: A controlled study. *Pediatrics, 65,* 948–955.

Vandvik, I.H. and Eckblad, G. (1991) Mothers of children with recent onset of rheumatic disease: Associations between maternal distress, psychosocial variables, and the disease of the children. *Developmental and Behavioural Pediatrics, 12,* 84–91.

Vanfossen, B.E. (1986) Sex differences in depression: The role of spouse support. In S.E. Hobfoll (ed.) *Stress, Social Support and Women.* Washington, D.C.: Hemisphere (pp. 69–83).

Varni, J.W. and Wallander, J.L. (1988) Pediatric chronic disabilities: Hemophilia and spina bifida as examples. In D. Routh (ed.) *Handbook of Pediatric Psychology.* New York: Guilford Press, pp.190–221.

Vaughn, B.E., Stevenson-Hinde, J., Waters, E., Kotsaftis, A., Lefever, G.B., Shouldice, A., Trudel, M. and Belsky, J. (1992) Attachment security and temperament in infancy and early childhood: Some conceptual clarifications. *Developmental Psychology, 28,* 463–473.

Vernon, D.T.A., Foley, J.M. and Schulman, J.L. (1967) Effect of mother–child separation and birth order on young children's responses to two potentially stressful situations. *Journal of Personality and Social Psychology, 5,* 162–174.

Voeller, K. and Rothenberg, M. (1973) Psychological aspects of the management of seizures in children. *Pediatrics, 51,* 1072–1082.

ᵩ Walker, C.L. (1988) Stress and coping in siblings of childhood cancer patients. *Nursing Research, 37,* 208–212.

Walker, D.K. (1984) Care of chronically ill children in schools. *Pediatric Clinics of North America, 31,* 221–233.

Walker, D.K., Stein, R.E.K., Perrin, E.C. and Jessop, D.J. (1990) Assessing psychosocial adjustment of children with chronic illnesses: A review of the technical properties of PARS III. *Journal of Developmental and Behavioural Pediatrics, 11,* 116–121.

ᵩ Walker, J.H., Thomas, M. and Russell, I.T. (1971) Spina Bifida – and the parents. *Developmental Medicine and Child Neurology, 13,* 462–476.

Walker, L.J. and Greene, J.W. (1991) The functional disability inventory: Measuring a neglected dimension of child health status. *Journal of Pediatric Psychology, 16,* 39–58.

Walker, L.S., Ford, M.B. and Donald, W.D. (1987) Cystic fibrosis and family stress: Effects of age and severity of illness. *Pediatrics, 79,* 239–246.

Walker, L.S., Ortiz-Valdes, J.A. and Newbrough, J.R. (1989) The role of maternal employment and depression in the psychological adjustment of chronically ill, mentally retarded and well children. *Journal of Pediatric Psychology, 14,* 357–370.

Wallander, J.L. and Hardy, D. (1991) Physically disabled adolescents: Coping with disability-related psychological problems. Unpublished data, University of Alabama at Birmingham.

Wallander, J.L., Varni, J.W., Babani, L., Banis, H.T., Wilcox, K.T. (1988) Children with chronic physical disorders: Maternal reports of their psychological adjustment. *Journal of Pediatric Psychology, 13,* 197–212.

Wallander, J.L., Varni, J.W., Babani, L., DeHeen, C.B., Wilcox, K.T. and Banis, H.T. (1989) The social environment and the adaptation of mothers of physically handicapped children. *Journal of Pediatric Psychology, 14,* 371–388.

Waller, D.A., Chipman, J.J., B.W., Hightower, M.J., North, A.J., Williams, J.B. and Babick, A.J. (1986) Measuring diabetes specific family support and its relation to metabolic control: a preliminary report. *Journal of the American Academy of Child Psychiatry, 25,* 415–418.

Walsh, J.K. (1985) Adolescent diabetes (A symposium held in March 1985). *Practical Diabetes, 2,* 20.

Ward, F. and Bower, B.D. (1978) A study of certain social aspects of epilepsy in childhood. *Developmental Medicine and Child Neurology, 20,* Supp. 39 (1–63).

Warne, J. (1988) Diabetes in school: a study of teachers' knowledge and information sources. *Practical Diabetes, 5,* 210–215.

Wasilewski, Y., Clark, N., Evans, D., Feldman, C.H., Kaplan, D., Rips, J. and Mellins, R.B. (1988) The effect of paternal social support on maternal disruption caused by childhood asthma. *Journal of Community Health, 13*, 33–42.

Wasserman, A.L., Thompson, E.L., Wilimas, J.A. and Fairclough, J. (1987) The psychological status of survivors of childhood/adolescent Hodgkin's disease. *Archives of Disease in Childhood, 141*, 636–31.

Wasserman, G.A. and Allen, R. (1985) Maternal withdrawal from handicapped toddlers. *Journal of Child Psychology and Psychiatry, 26*, 381–387.

Waters, E. and Deane, K.E. (1985) Defining and assessing individual differences in infant attachment relationships: Q-methodology and the organization of behaviour. In I. Bretherton and E. Waters (eds.) *Growing Pains of Attachment Theory and Research. Monographs of the Society of Research in Child Development, 50*, (Serial No. 209) (pp.41–65).

Webster-Stratton, C. (1990) Stress: A potential disrupter of parent perceptions and family interactions. *Journal of Clinical Child Psychology, 19*, 302–312.

Weiland, S.K., Pless, I.B. and Roghmann, K.J. (1992) Chronic illness and mental health problems in pediatric practice: Results from a survey of primary care providers. *Pediatrics, 89*, 445–449.

Weinberger, M., Cohen, S.J. and Mazzuca, S.A. (1984) The role of physicians' knowledge and attitudes in effective diabetes management. *Social Science and Medicine, 19*, 965–969.

Weinstein, A.G. and Cuskey, W. (1985) Theophylline compliance in asthmatic children. *Annuals Allergy, 54*, 19–24.

Weitzman, M. (1984) School and peer relations. *Pediatric Clinics of North America, 31*, 59–69.

Weitzman, M. (1986) School absence rates as outcome measures in studies of children with chronic illnesses. *Journal of Chronic Disease, 39*, 799–808.

Wertlieb, D., Hauser, S.T. and Jacobson, A. (1986) Adaptation to diabetes: Behaviour symptoms and family context. *Journal of Pediatric Psychology, 11*, 463–480.

Whitt, J.K., Dykstra, W. and Taylor, C.A. (1979) Children's conceptions of illness and cognitive development. *Clinical Pediatrics, 18*, 327–339.

Wiley, F.M., Lindamood, M.M. and Pfefferbaum-Levine, B. (1984) Donor–patient relationship in pediatric bone-marrow transplantation *Journal of Association of Pediatric Oncology Nurses, 1*, 8–14.

Willis, D.J., Elliott, C.H. and Jay, S.M. (1982) Psychological effects of physical illness and its concomitants. In J. Tuma (ed.) *Handbook for the Practice of Pediatric Psychology*, New York: Wiley (pp.28–66).

Wolfer, J.A. and Wisintainer, M.A. (1979) Prehospital psychological preparation for tonsillectomy patients: Effects on children's and parents' adjustment. *Pediatrics, 64*, 646–655.

Woolf, A., Rappaport, L., Reardon, P., Ciborowski, J., D'Angelo, E. and Bessette, J. (1989) School functioning and disease severity in boys with hemophilia. *Journal of Developmental and Behavioural Pediatrics, 10*, 81–85.

Wortman, C.B. and Silver, R.C (1987) Coping with irrevocable loss. In G.R. VandenBos and B.K. Bryant (eds.) *Cataclysms, Crises and Catastrophes.* Washington, D.C.: APA. (pp.185–235).

Wysocki, T., Meinhold, P., Abrams, K., Barnard, M., Clarke, W.L., Bellando, J. and Bourgeois, M. (in press). Parental and professional estimates of self-care independence of children and adolescents with insulin-dependent diabetes mellitus. *Diabetes Care.*

Wysocki, T., Meinhold, P., Cos, D.J. and Clarke, W.L. (1990) Survey of diabetes professionals regarding development changes in diabetes self-care. *Diabetes Care, 13,* 65–58.

Yoak, M., Chesney, B.K. and Schartz, N.H. (1985) Active roles in self-help groups for parents of children with cancer. *Childrens' Health Care, 14,* 38–45.

Zabin, M. and Melamed, B.G. (1980) The relationship between parental discipline and children's ability to cope with stress. *Journal of Behavioural Assessment, 2,* 17–38.

Zastowny, T.R., Kirschenbaum, D.S. and Meng, A.L. (1986) Coping skills training for children: Effects on distress before, during, and after hospitalization for surgery. *Health Psychology, 5,* 231–247.

Zrebiec, J.F. (1987) Psychosocial commentary on insulin-dependent diabetes mellitus in 5- to 9-year-old children. In S.J. Brink (ed.) *Pediatric and Adolescent Diabetes Mellitus.* Chicago: Year Book Medical Publishers (pp.79–88).

Subject Index

Name Index